THE
ULTIMATE
DIET
BOOK

Slimming
MAGAZINE

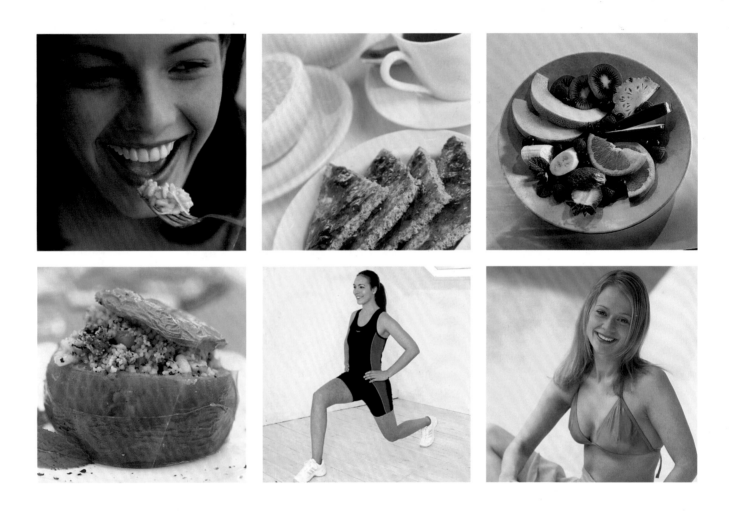

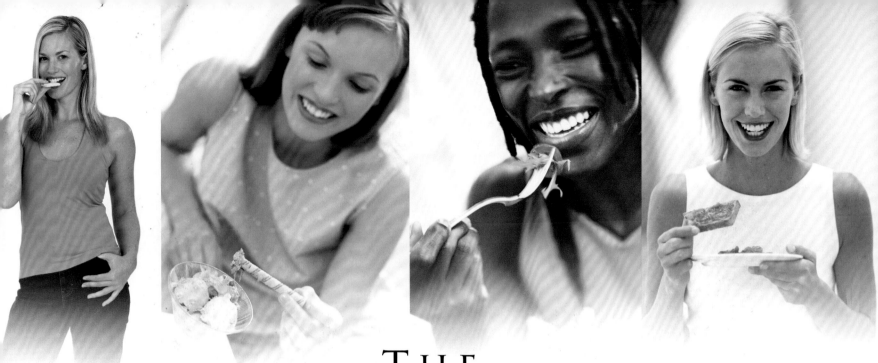

THE
ULTIMATE
DIET
BOOK

Slimming
MAGAZINE

First published in 2003

A catalogue record for this book is available from the British Library

ISBN 1 84425 143 8

Published jointly by
Haynes Publishing, Sparkford,
Yeovil, Somerset BA22 7JJ, England
Phone 01963 440635, www.haynes.co.uk
And
Emap Esprit Limited,
Wentworth House, Wentworth Street,
Peterborough PE1 1DS, England
Phone 01733 213700, www.emap.com

Printed and bound in England by J.H. Haynes & Co. Ltd, Sparkford

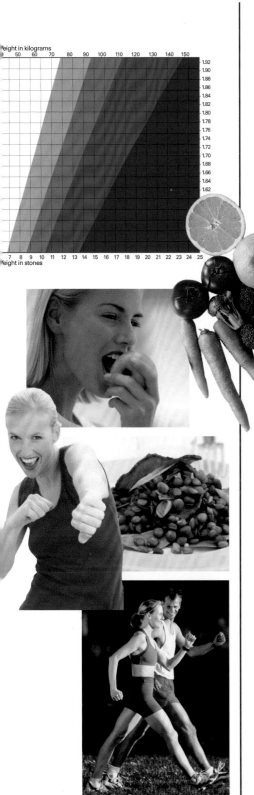

CONTENTS

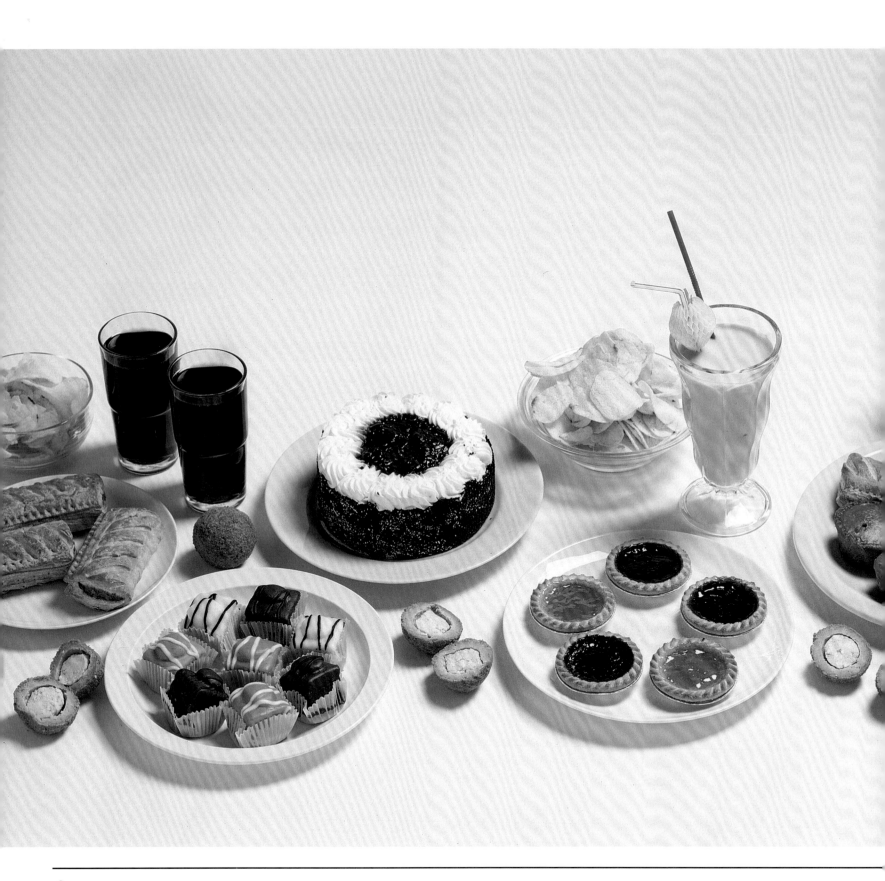

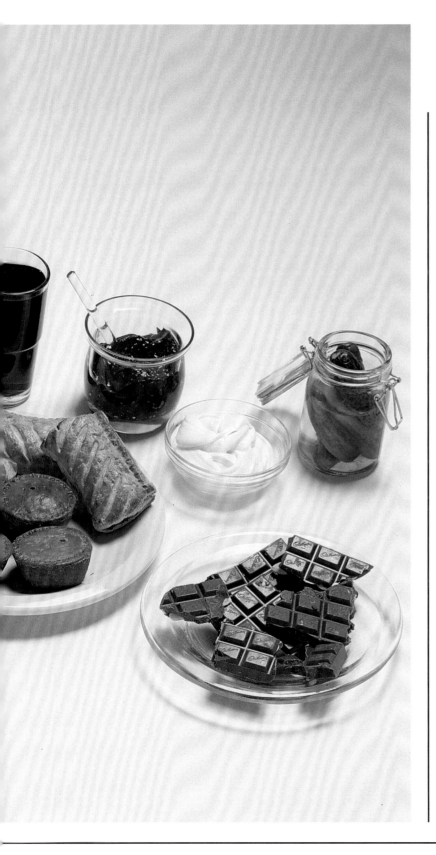

Foreword
by Rashmi Madan

Editor of Slimming Magazine

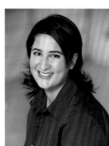

Our lifestyles and diets have changed drastically over the past ten years and for the first time ever, more people in the world are officially overweight or obese than those who are of normal weight or underweight. It's become common place to 'go on a diet'. It's also more acceptable - thanks to all the celebrities who openly reveal their weight-loss secrets (although the majority are on faddy eating plans). This book has something for everyone - a variety of different diets (to keep you from getting bored) for people with less than a stone, between 1st and 3st and with more than 3st to lose. There are exercise routines for beginners to workouts for advanced gym goers and what's more, there are lots of inspiring real-life success stories to help motivate you along the way. Diets won't fail you - as long as you follow the advice given and stick to it, you will lose weight. Add some regular exercise three to five times a week and you have a recipe for success. Remember, a safe weight loss of 1lb-2lb a week is the best way to keep weight off. So, what are you waiting for? This book will help you be the shape you want. Good luck!

The publishers would like to acknowledge the diligent efforts of Susan Voss and the staff of Emap Licensing for making this project possible.

HEIGHT		WEIGHT RANGE				
Ft	in	St	lb	to	St	lb
4	11	7	1		8	12
5	0	7	5		9	3
5	1	7	8		9	7
5	2	7	12		9	11
5	3	8	1		10	1
5	4	8	4		10	5
5	5	8	8		10	10
5	6	8	12		11	1
5	7	9	2		11	6
5	8	9	6		11	11
5	9	9	10		12	2
5	10	10	0		12	7
5	11	10	4		12	12
6	0	10	8		13	3

The help

The new slimline you, just a healthy diet away, doesn't have to be a skinny bean, because there's no single, ideal weight for everyone. To stay fit and feel good, you should weigh a healthy weight for your height. Nutrition experts agree that there is a healthy weight range (see the chart, right), and that people outside this will be more prone to health problems like diabetes, heart disease, high blood pressure, certain cancers, gallstones or joint and back problems. Within the range, find the weight at which you feel and look best. Don't aim below the healthy weight for your height, though – it's just as unhealthy to be underweight, as you may not be eating enough to get all the nutrients you need.

How much can I expect to lose?

Follow a diet and you should lose 1lb to 2lb a week. It may be a little more when you first start your diet due to a loss of water as well as fat. But if you regularly lose more than this you'll be losing muscle, too. Follow our guidelines for slow and steady weight loss:
- Eat a variety of different foods
- Eat lots of foods rich in starch and fibre
- Don't eat too much fat or sugar
- Get the right balance of essential vitamins and minerals
- Keep within sensible alcohol limits

▼ This chart – for men and women – is based on the Body Mass Index (BMI), a way of estimating healthy weight now used widely by GPs.

Body mass index chart

CALCULATING YOUR BMI
Another way to find out if you're over- or underweight is to work out your BMI by dividing your weight in kilograms by your height in metres squared. For example, if you're 5ft 4in and 11st, convert your height into metres and your weight into kilograms: 1.63m and 70kg respectively. Then square your height: 1.63 x 1.63 = 2.66. Finally, divide your weight by your height squared, eg 70 ÷ 2.66 = 26.3. Your ideal BMI should be between 20 and 25.

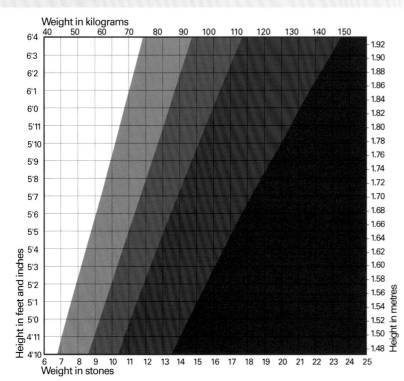

UNDERWEIGHT (BMI UNDER 20)
You may need to eat more to gain weight. Choose starchy foods, fruit and vegetables.

NORMAL WEIGHT (BMI 20 TO 25)
Keep your weight steady and don't be tempted to aim for the underweight category. If your weight has been creeping up, take action now so that you don't become overweight.

OVERWEIGHT (BMI 25 TO 30)
Avoid gaining more weight and concentrate on losing 1lb to 2lb a week.

VERY OVERWEIGHT (BMI 30 TO 40)
It's essential to lose weight and even a loss of 1st will benefit your health.

SERIOUSLY OVERWEIGHT (BMI MORE THAN 40)
Your health is seriously at risk so you must lose weight. Ask your GP for advice.

This scale is suitable for both men and women, but not for growing children or teenagers, pregnant women or sportsmen and women with a high proportion of muscle, which weighs more than fat.

centre

Want to get in shape? All the information you need to lose weight the healthy way is right here

What's the best way to lose weight?

You can either count calories or the number of fat grams you eat each day

CALORIE COUNTING

Calories are a measure of the energy content of foods. Eat more calories than you need and you gain weight. Have fewer calories than you need and you'll lose weight. The calories you need each day to keep your weight steady depends on your height, age and the amount of exercise you do. Women need approximately 2,000 calories a day and men need approximately 2,500.

One pound of fat contains 3,500 calories. So to lose 1lb in a week you need to eat 3,500 fewer calories. You can do this by cutting 500 calories a day from the 2,000 (average amount of calories for women) you need to maintain your weight. But experts now believe that the healthiest way to diet is to lose those 500 calories through a combination of eating less and exercising regularly.

To find out how many calories you need to be eating each day, see the values below. The figures assume that you're exercising for 30 minutes three to fives time a week. If you're not exercising this frequently (but we recommend that you do, as it will boost your metabolism and tone your body), you need to eat 250 calories less a day than shown.

■ Women under 30 may need 100 calories and 3g to 4g more fat per day than shown.

■ Women aged 60 or over may need 200 calories and 6g to 8g less fat per day than shown.

■ Values not for children under 18.

Fat grams are important, too. If you're counting calories, for healthy weight loss you need to watch your fat intake, too. You could lose weight on 1,500 calories worth of chocolate bars a day, but you'd be getting too much fat and missing essential nutrients.

As a nation we're getting over 40% of our calories from fat. This is too high: the Department of Health says this should be 33%. For weight loss 25% to 30% of your daily calories should come from fat. The table shows how many grams of fat you need depending on your calorie allowance. To monitor your intake use food labels as a guide. For every 100 calories, the food should have no more than 3g fat; for 200 calories, no more than 6g, and so on.

Here's what you're allowed

WEIGHT TO LOSE	AVERAGE CALS DAILY		FAT GRAMS DAILY 25-30%	25-30%	ALCOHOL UNITS PER WEEK	
	Women	Men	Women	Men	Women	Men
Less than 1st	1,250	1,500	35-42g	42-50g	2.5	3
1st to 3st	1,500	1,750	42-50g	49-58g	3	3.5
More than 3st	1,800	2,050	50-60g	57-68g	3.5	4

COUNTING FAT GRAMS

This suits people with big appetites. Because fat has so many calories, avoiding it where possible while still having generous amounts of carbohydrates and low-fat protein will help you lose weight without counting calories. This means you can fill up on low-fat foods, such as rice, but will still lose weight if you're eating larger portions than calorie counters. Cutting back on fat doesn't mean no fat. You need some fat to be healthy; aim to cut back on the saturated kind. While you can eat unlimited amounts of virtually fat-free foods, some sugary foods are low-fat but high-calorie, so eat low-sugar alternatives. And although most alcohol is fat-free, it's high in calories, so stick to the units shown above (one unit = 275ml/½pt bitter, lager or cider; a single pub measure of spirits; or a small glass of wine or sherry).

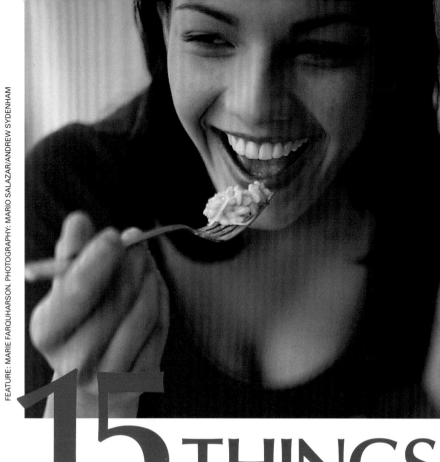

FEATURE: MARIE FARQUHARSON. PHOTOGRAPHY: MARIO SALAZAR/ANDREW SYDENHAM

15 THINGS
you must know to lose weight

Why do late nights make you eat more and why shouldn't you miss breakfast? Understanding the key weight-loss factors could make all the difference to your diet

3 Get enough protein

WHY THIS WORKS: Protein fills you up faster and helps you stay fuller for longer than either fats or carbs. Some experts believe it's because proteins take longer to break down, while others claim that when proteins are digested they trigger the hormones that make you feel full. Aim to eat a little protein at each meal.

Carbohydrate-only meals push up your insulin levels, which triggers your appetite. Adding protein to your meals will help balance blood sugar levels and curb hunger pangs, and prevent fatigue. Aim to get between 15% to 20% of your total calories from protein. Opt for lean meats, fish, beans and low-fat dairy products.

4 Believe you can lose the weight

WHY THIS WORKS: Studies continue to show that people who lose weight and keep it off believe that they can make it happen.

To muster up that self-belief, spend a few quiet minutes every day visualising why you want to lose weight. For example, picture yourself in a summer frock, playing with your kids, or feeling fitter and healthier.

5 Allow yourself the occasional treat

WHY THIS WORKS: It seems a good idea to skip desserts, chocolate, cakes and all your favourite treats until you hit your ideal weight. But denying yourself certain foods will, in most cases, backfire, as it only leads to you feeling deprived. 'If you tell yourself not to think of pink elephants, you'll find it pretty hard to shift that image from your mind,' says Pete Cohen, creator of the Lighten Up Programme. The same applies when you tell yourself you're never going to eat biscuits again. Suddenly they become the very thing you crave. No foods are off limits: just eat a little of what you fancy and leave it at that.

1 Eat enough calories

WHY THIS WORKS: Very low-calorie diets slow down your metabolism, encouraging your body to hold onto what little food you're giving it. This will make it harder to lose weight as well as upping your risk of gallstones and gout. You'll feel hungry and deprived, give up on the diet and be more likely to binge later on.

2 Trim the fat from your diet

WHY THIS WORKS: Weight for weight, fat has more calories (9 per gram) than protein or carbs (both 4 calories per gram), and it's less bulky, so it's easier to overeat. The key word is trim the fat, not cut. A small amount is vital for your body to absorb fat-soluble vitamins, such as A and E. Try to get 25% to 30% of your calories from fat, mainly from vegetable sources such as olive, sunflower and peanut oil.

6 Set yourself realistic goals

WHY THIS WORKS: You may be hell-bent on dropping three dress sizes before your sister's wedding in September but the healthiest way to get there is to focus on small, achievable short-term goals, according to studies conducted at the University of Pennsylvania School of Medicine. Researchers found that obese men and women who set themselves a modest goal of losing just 5% to 10% of their body weight are more likely to succeed than those who set more demanding goals. This is because long-term goals can seem too distant to inspire you to make healthy choices dozens of times a day. Also, focusing on the larger picture of, say, wanting to lose 3st can devalue the achievement of the 2lb you've shifted this week.

Your short-term goals could be: to lose between 1lb to 2lb a week, to stick to your healthy eating plan, or to work out three times a week.

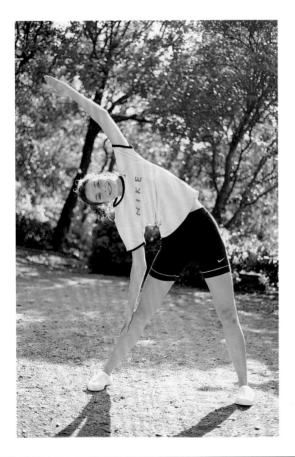

7 Eat more slowly

WHY THIS WORKS: It takes about 20 minutes for your body to register that you feel full. By eating too quickly you may scoff far more than you need before you receive the signal to stop.

Pace yourself by putting down your knife and fork between bites, and hold off loading up your fork until you've finished your current mouthful. As you chew, savour the flavour and texture of your food.

8 Exercise regularly

WHY THIS WORKS: The more exercise you do, the more calories you burn and the more fat you lose. And studies have found that when you exercise your brain releases the feel-good hormone serotonin, which suppresses hunger. For weight loss, exercise for 20 to 30 minutes three to five times a week, building in both aerobic and strength or weight training sessions. Doing both cardio and resistance work burns more fat than doing either type of exercise on its own.

9 Eat fibre

WHY THIS WORKS: Fibre fills you up quickly so you don't overeat and takes longer to digest so you stay full for longer. Get your fibre from wholegrains (brown rice, porridge oats, wholewheat pasta), root vegetables (such as potatoes), pulses and fruit. Up your intake slowly, and drink plenty of water to flush it out.

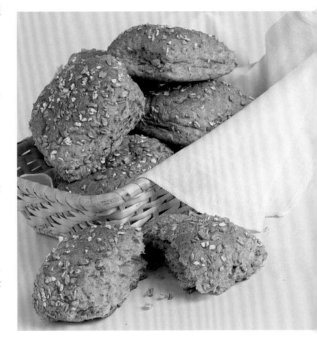

10 Drink up

WHY THIS WORKS: If you don't drink enough water it can leave you dehydrated, tired and unable to think clearly. It's also easy to confuse thirst for hunger and eat something, when what you really need is a large glass of water. Aim to drink at least eight glasses of water a day.

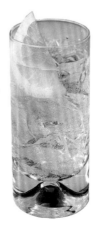

11 Watch your portion sizes

WHY THIS WORKS: When you eat too much food your body has to deal with the excess. Eat too much protein and your body will store it first as glucose for energy; if it's not needed, the glucose will be converted into fat. Excess carbohydrates are converted into fat, as is any excess fat that you eat. So whatever way you look at it, if you overpile your plate or tuck into a snack when you're not hungry the result is the same: the calories your body has no use for are stored as fat – and you'll put on weight. Watch your portions and the weight will come off.

12 Get your calcium

WHY THIS WORKS: You know that calcium is vital for strong bones and to protect against osteoporosis (brittle bones). But did you know this mineral can help you lose weight? Upping your calcium intake when you're on a diet has been linked to increased weight loss in a study at the University of Vermont. Of the 181 women who took part in the study, those who increased their calcium intake by 130mg a day (the amount found in just over ¼pt skimmed milk) lost more weight than those who didn't. And it seems that getting 1,000mg calcium a day may shift the pounds even faster. One explanation for this comes from a team of researchers studying human fat cells: 'If you don't get enough calcium your body releases a hormone that draws the mineral from your bones. The same hormone directs fat cells to store more fat,' says Michael Zemel, professor of Nutrition and Medicine at the University of Tennessee. Good sources of calcium include: reduced-fat Cheddar (840mg calcium per 100g); sardines and their bones, canned in brine, drained (540mg per 100g); almonds (240mg per 100g), low-fat yoghurt (190mg per 100g); haricot beans (180mg per 100g, dry weight); chickpeas (160mg per 100g, dry weight); and white bread, skimmed and semi-skimmed milk (all 120mg per 100g).

13 Get plenty of sleep

WHY THIS WORKS: You eat more when you're tired. A lack of sleep can make you feel you're running on empty, so you're more likely to crave sugary foods. Plus, staying up late encourages your body to produce more of the stress hormone cortisol. It's largely responsible for waking you up in the morning but at night raised cortisol levels trigger cravings for fatty and starchy foods. To add insult to injury, cortisol also encourages your body to store fat. To get a good night's sleep, set yourself a regular bedtime and stick to it even on your days off, take a warm – not hot – bath to help you relax and avoid exercising within three hours of bedtime, to give your body a chance to wind down.

14 Eat a good breakfast

WHY THIS WORKS: Missing breakfast in an attempt to save calories for later can set you up to overeat for the rest of the day. After having 'fasted' all night, your blood sugar levels will be low. Miss breakfast and you'll find it harder to resist sweet, fatty snacks later in the morning. For a good-size breakfast try: two slices of wholemeal toast with 1tsp peanut butter and a small banana (275 calories and 5.9g fat), or a bowl of muesli with skimmed milk and a kiwi fruit (252 calories and 3.1g fat).

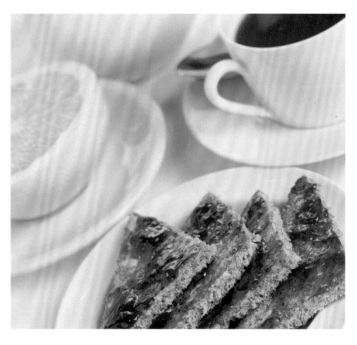

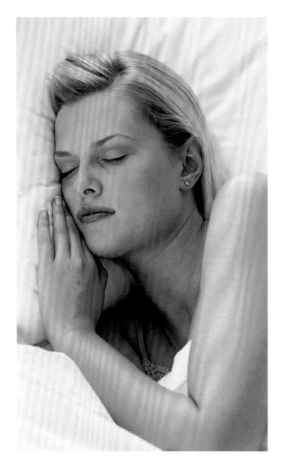

15 Develop a plan

WHY THIS WORKS: You'll avoid slipping into 'old' eating habits. Try these tricks to keep you focused:

• Keep a food diary. It will help you to recognise any self-defeating patterns you may have developed.

• Learn from your failures but don't stew in them. Acknowledge, then move on.

• Do take responsibility. Deep down you know your typical excuses. Now's the time to ditch them and find solutions.

• Plan your goals. Make them specific and challenging but realistic, and remember to celebrate your achievements.

• Know what motivates you, be open to new influences and look for inspiration.

7 steps to becoming a smart shopper

One moment of weakness in the supermarket can lead to a trolley-full of stodge, but shop smartly and you'll leave the store with all the ingredients for a healthy week ahead

FEATURE: LARA KILNER
PHOTOGRAPHY: ANDREW SYDENHAM

1 Stock up

Never, ever go to buy food when you're hungry – it's the number one rule of grocery shopping. Going to the supermarket when you're feeling peckish, never mind ravenous, is only going to end in a cream bun-filled trolley. The best time to go is after a meal – ideally in the morning after breakfast, so that you're full, fresh, alert and more likely to make the most diet-friendly decisions on what to buy.

2 Be prepared

Write a shopping list – and don't deviate from it. Plan a week's worth of healthy meals in advance and keep it varied so you don't get bored. If you've got exactly what you need to buy written down, you're less likely to go haywire and end up filling the trolley with bumper-sized packs of muffins.

3 It's all in the label

Become a slave to labels, taking heed of the calorie and saturated fat content. Be wary of foods labelled 'reduced fat' – they can have more calories than the regular brands because of their increased sugar content. OK, so your shopping might take twice as long, but at least you'll know what you're putting in your mouth at the end of it.

4 You're kidding

Most kids don't reckon their lunch boxes are complete without gallons of fizzy pop and packets of crisps. Your life might not be worth living if you omit these essentials, but don't buy them at the supermarket – give them tuck shop money or grab them at the local shop before the school run. If these foods aren't lingering in your kitchen cupboards, you can't succumb to their allure.

5 Be aisle savvy

Always start with the fresh produce section. Fill your trolley with fresh fruit and veg, so you won't have room for those family-sized tins of biscuits, even if you want them. And remember, many of the more tempting foods will be bunched together, so don't go down the aisles that aren't relevant to you. And by that, we mean those playing host to the dreaded 'C's – chocolate, crisps, cakes – you know the rest...

6 Maximise your nutrients

In the produce section, opt for dark green veg (the darker the colour, the more vitamins and minerals). Ditch nutrient-free iceberg lettuce in favour of iron-packed watercress. Opt for wholegrains in favour of refined carbohydrates – which means wholemeal bread or wholewheat pasta in place of white. Darker foods contain more fibre, folic acid, zinc and magnesium. Opt for oily fish, which contains fatty acids to keep your heart healthy and, dairy wise, cut the high-fat options like butter and replace full-fat milk with skimmed – it has the same amount of calcium. And don't dismiss the frozen section – freshly frozen veg is often as nutritious as its fresh neighbour.

7 Go solo

If you're planning to stay focused and on track, do you really want that pesky family of yours on hand? No doubt hubby will be sneaking four packs of lager and microwave curries in the trolley to his heart's content, and the kiddies will be screaming for bumper bags of calorie-laden sweets. Going it alone is the most diet-friendly option.

5 REASONS for OVEREATING

It's easy to overeat without realising you're doing it. Here are our tips on beating the munchies

You know that to lose weight you need to eat fewer calories than your body needs. But it's not always that simple, is it? Even with the best intentions in the world, it's easy to stray from your diet and have an extra slice of cake or another biscuit. So figuring out just why you overeat is crucial to tackling the habit and learning how to break free of it – once and for all. We show you how...

1 OVEREATING BECAUSE YOU'RE TIRED

Why does it happen?
Most people overeat when they're tired for two reasons. Firstly, if you haven't had enough sleep you probably snack on high-sugar foods like cakes and chocolate for a quick energy boost during the day. Secondly, if you're working late or staying up past the time you normally go to bed, eating can often be a way to distract yourself to keep awake.

Why is this a bad idea?
When you snack through tiredness you might think you're giving yourself an energy boost, but you could leave yourself more tired than before. Why? It's all down to what you eat. Gillan Riley, addiction therapist, says, 'too often, you probably reach for stimulants such as coffee, chocolate and sugar for a short energy rush. But this is followed by an energy slump, leaving you more tired'.

How to sort it
● It's fine to snack when you're tired, just choose foods that give you longer-lasting energy, like a wholemeal scone or banana sandwiched between slices of wholemeal bread, and include it in your calorie allowance.

● Try exercising to energise you – even a quick walk outside can wake you up.

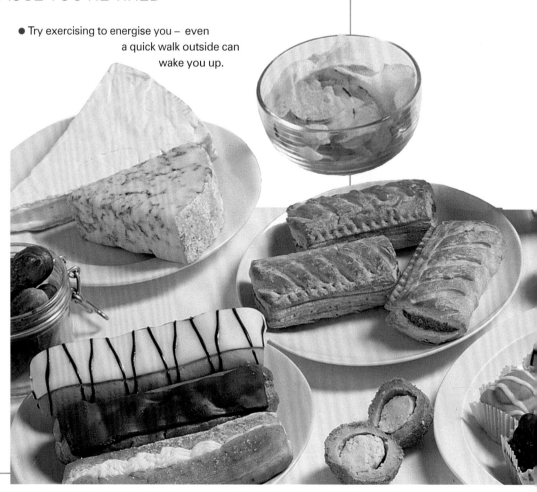

2 OVEREATING BECAUSE YOU'RE UPSET OR BORED

Why does it happen?

'People often overeat when they're upset or bored because of the "diversion factor",' says Catherine Collins of the British Dietetic Association. We temporarily take our minds off whatever the problem is – whether it's a row with a loved one, work stress, frustration at being home alone with nothing to do – by giving ourselves a 'treat' of food.

Gillian Riley takes this further. 'Over time, eating when you're upset or bored becomes a habit – people do it because they've done it in the past. Remember the scientist Pavlov's experiment? He'd ring a bell and then give dogs some food. Eventually, the dogs salivated at the sound of the bell, without there being any food. We can end up conditioning ourselves in a similar way and eating when we feel down because it's what we're used to.'

Why is this a bad idea?

Overeating when you're upset or bored doesn't improve the situation, and the extra weight gain will just make you feel worse about yourself. It can also leave you feeling that everything in your life is somehow out of control.

How to sort it

- Learn that you have a choice. If you want a tub of ice cream when you're upset or bored, you can have it – but accept that you're choosing to eat it and that, calorie-wise, you might regret it afterwards. By making decisions around food more consciously, you'll start to break away from your conditioned pattern of eating when you're upset, and separate eating from emotions.

- Acknowledge that you're upset or bored rather than hungry. When you're tempted to reach for that chocolate bar, ask yourself if it's really what will help you feel better.
- Try to pinpoint the things that are making you upset, or ask yourself why you're bored, and take action. If you feel your boss undermines you, think about going on an assertiveness training course to learn to stand up for yourself. If you're stuck at home all day with nothing to do but eat, find a new hobby to occupy you.

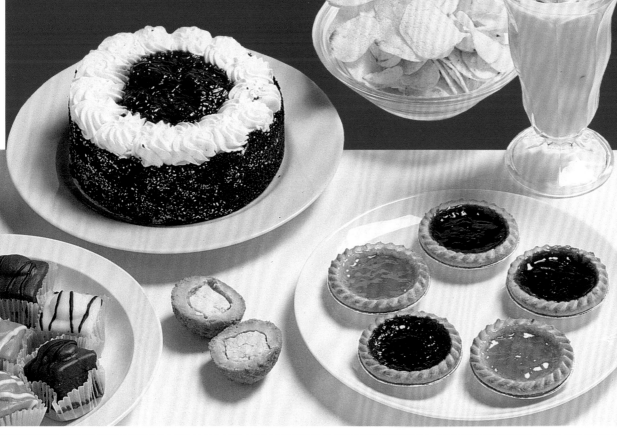

3 OVEREATING BECAUSE YOU GRAZE THOUGHOUT THE DAY

Why does it happen?
These days, we have less time for ourselves and don't take proper lunch breaks. 'If people work in an office, they do something else while they're eating, like surf the internet,' Catherine Collins says. 'Parents eat on the run while chasing around after their kids. All these things mean that people are less likely to register what they've eaten, so it's more likely that they'll overeat later.'

Another time you might not realise you overeat is when you're standing up. 'It happens a lot when you're preparing a meal in the kitchen,' says Catherine. 'You have easy access to cupboards and fridge doors and often there are packets of food at eye level.' Eating food from children's plates when you're clearing away, telling yourself you 'mustn't waste it', is another way of having extra calories.

Why is this a bad idea?
'Grazing in itself isn't a bad thing,' says Gillian Riley. 'If you graze on fruit or salad, you don't have a problem. The difficulties start if you're going for high-sugar options. Eating junk food means that you develop a taste for it, and can become less inclined to choose healthier options.'

And eating while you're standing up can be a bad idea because you don't recognise how many calories you're taking on board. Also, you may not count the calories as you don't recognise it as a meal. 'When I get people to keep food diaries, they're often amazed by how much they're eating without noticing – this tends not to be particularly enjoyable eating, so it would be far more sensible for them to save those calories to consume during a proper meal.'

How to sort it
● If you have to graze, choose healthy options like fruit or raw vegetables.
● Plan your grazing so you can include it in your calorie allowance, instead of eating unaware. Or keep track of the calories you have by keeping a food diary and writing down everything you eat or drink.
● Have something in your mouth when you cook, to help you resist snacking. Chewing gum is perfect.
● Bin the children's leftovers straightaway. That way, the food won't be hanging around waiting for you to pick at it.

4 OVEREATING BECAUSE YOU KEEP ON EATING EVEN AFTER YOU'RE FULL

Why does it happen?
People carry on eating when they're full for all sorts of reasons. Maybe you grew up in a family where everyone had second or third helpings and it's become a habit. Or perhaps your children have left home but you're still preparing the same amounts of food – and eating it yourself. Another reason could be that when you're socialising you eat more than you need to just because everyone else is.

Why is it a bad idea?
Continuing to eat when you're full can leave you feeling bloated and uncomfortable. And by keeping going, all you're doing is increasing your calorie intake. As a result, if you're on a diet you might need to cut back on calories – to keep within your allowance – at a time when you really are hungry. So don't make it harder on yourself just because you're not thinking.

How to sort it
● Decide how much you want to eat

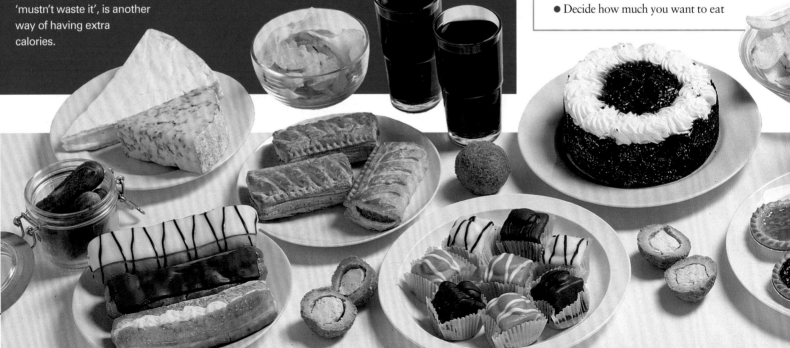

before you sit down to a meal. When you've finished that amount, accept that you'll probably feel you could eat more. But if you slow down and ask yourself whether you're really still hungry, you'll find you can stop.

● Watch your second helpings. Cook extra veg with your meals – then if you want a second helping, make sure it's just vegetables.

● Listen to your stomach. Remember that it takes 20 minutes for your brain to register that your stomach is full. If you wait a while after you've eaten your meal, chances are you won't actually feel like having another plateful.

● Chew your food slowly and get the most from each mouthful. This will slow down the rate at which you eat, and you'll appreciate the flavour of your food more.

● Get used to saying 'no' when people try to feed you extra portions. Some of them might not like the thought of you getting slimmer – maybe your partner's worried that you'll find someone else if you're slim. Reassure them you just want to lead a healthy lifestyle.

● Have fruit as dessert. That way, you won't feel as if you're missing out on a pudding. If you do have dessert, just have a smaller portion.

5 OVEREATING BECAUSE YOU'RE NOT ORGANISED

Why does it happen?

'Our work environments are getting more demanding,' says Catherine Collins. 'Work often takes priority over everything else, and we don't have time to organise our home life.' Maybe you get home in the evening to find that you don't have anything low fat in the fridge, and then defrost a high-calorie pizza or order a takeaway. Or you end up bingeing on the high-fat snacks at the back of the cupboard when there's nothing else to eat.

Why is this a bad idea?

Overeating because you're not organised can leave you feeling chaotic and bad about yourself. You're also giving yourself the message that your health and wellbeing are at the bottom of your list of priorities – which isn't good for your self-esteem. Not to mention the fact that constantly eating takeaways can be hard on your wallet, and uses up money that could be better spent giving yourself non-food-related treats like make-up or a massage.

How to sort it

● Stock up on low-fat foods – try buying frozen veg so you always have it in, and keep a supply of calorie-counted ready meals in the freezer for days when you're too tired to cook. When you do cook, make bigger portions and freeze some for other days.

● Plan meals in advance. If you know what you're going to eat, you can buy food at the start of the week and will have no excuse to dial for a takeaway when there's nothing else in the fridge.

● Limit the high-fat snacks you buy. Go supermarket shopping without your kids so they won't pester you to put extra biscuits or snacks in the trolley.

10 ways to speed up your metabolism

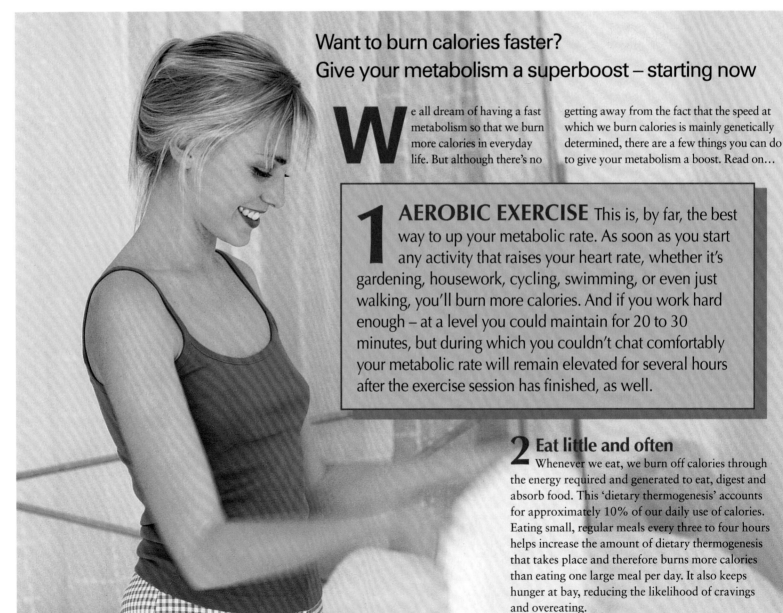

Want to burn calories faster?
Give your metabolism a superboost – starting now

We all dream of having a fast metabolism so that we burn more calories in everyday life. But although there's no getting away from the fact that the speed at which we burn calories is mainly genetically determined, there are a few things you can do to give your metabolism a boost. Read on…

1 AEROBIC EXERCISE This is, by far, the best way to up your metabolic rate. As soon as you start any activity that raises your heart rate, whether it's gardening, housework, cycling, swimming, or even just walking, you'll burn more calories. And if you work hard enough – at a level you could maintain for 20 to 30 minutes, but during which you couldn't chat comfortably your metabolic rate will remain elevated for several hours after the exercise session has finished, as well.

2 Eat little and often
Whenever we eat, we burn off calories through the energy required and generated to eat, digest and absorb food. This 'dietary thermogenesis' accounts for approximately 10% of our daily use of calories. Eating small, regular meals every three to four hours helps increase the amount of dietary thermogenesis that takes place and therefore burns more calories than eating one large meal per day. It also keeps hunger at bay, reducing the likelihood of cravings and overeating.

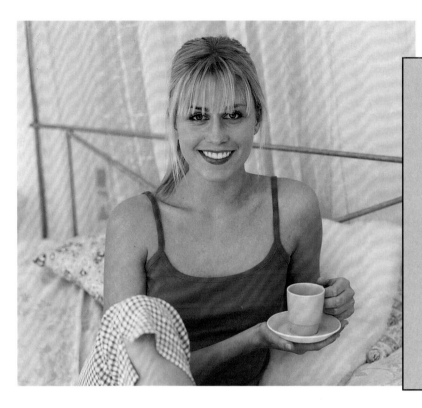

7 GO GREEN A Swiss study found that people who drink green tea burned significantly more calories than those that don't. It is thought that the phytochemical flavanoids found in the tea may affect the 'energy' hormone noradrenalanie which in turn, may speed up the rate at which fat is burned in the body. Green tea is also extremely good for overall health – it is thought to be a powerful antioxidant that helps boost the body's immune system – but again, because of the caffeine content, stick to a maximum of three to four cups a day.

3 Eat enough protein

Protein foods require up to 18% more energy to be digested than carbohydrates or fats, so make sure you're getting the recommended 15% of calories from protein. Government guidelines describe this as two to three servings of dairy products plus two to three servings of meat, fish, nuts, beans, or pulses a day. But don't go overboard, as too much protein can strain your kidneys and liver, and is also linked to loss of bone calcium and high blood pressure.

4 Spice up your life

Clinical research studies have found that an ingredient known as capsaicin found in spices, particularly chilli, can raise the metabolic rate by up to 50% for as long as three hours after a meal. This is because the heart rate increases when spices are eaten. Spices are great for flavouring low-fat dishes and they're good for you, too – capsaicin has anti-inflammatory properties and can help with conditions such as arthritis. Use enough chilli to make the meal spicy. Try adding chilli powder, chilli sauce, or fresh chillies to curries, fajitas, rice and pasta dishes, and stir-fries.

5 Give yourself a caffeine kick

Several studies have shown that as little as two and a half cups of coffee or a couple of cans of cola a day can raise the metabolism by 10% to 30% for one to three hours after drinking. (Go for diet colas though, as regular cola has, on average, 130 calories per can.) The caffeine found in both drinks increases your heart rate and the circulating amounts of the hormone adrenaline. However, more than three or four cups of coffee and two cans of coke aren't good for your general health, leading to agitation, insomnia and upset stomachs.

6 Eat your greens

To ensure the health of your thyroid, and particularly if there's a history of thyroid problems in your family, enrich your diet with sea greens such as dulse, kombu, wakame, or seafood. These contain iodine, which improves the function of the thyroid gland. This in turn may help raise the metabolic rate by increasing the production of thyroxin, which is the hormone responsible for regulating metabolism.

8 Get moving

A recent study in the US found that people who naturally fidget and move around burn up to 400 calories a day more than the rest of us. The researchers labelled this factor NEAT (non-exercise activity thermogenesis). If you're not a natural fidgeter you can burn the same amount of calories and more by increasing the activity in your life. Go for walks in your tea breaks, take the stairs and use your bike instead of the car whenever you can.

9 Turn down the heating

Try turning down the thermostat in your home or office by just a few degrees. This will force the body to burn more calories so that it can stay at its preferred temperature of 37°C.

10 Do strength training

It might not work overnight, but strength training (working muscles against a resistance sufficient to ensure you can't do more than 12 repetitions) is still one of the most effective ways to increase your metabolic rate. In fact, you'll burn an extra 50 calories a day for every 1lb of muscle tissue you put on. Consequently, regular strength training can increase your metabolic rate by as much as 15%.

6 WAYS to stop OBSESSING! (It could be making you fat)

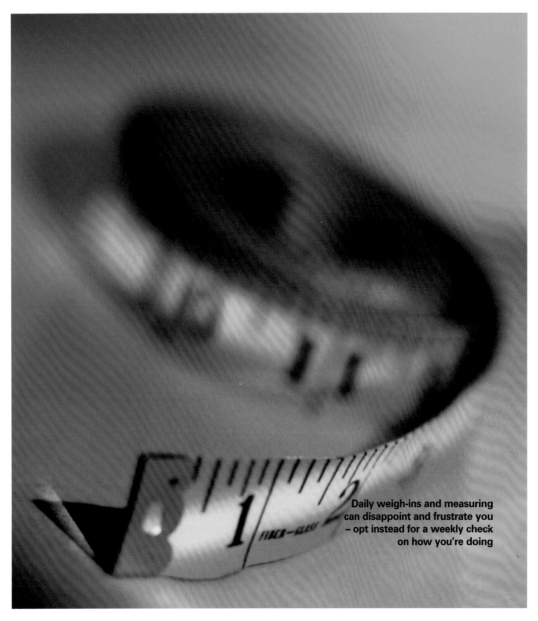

Daily weigh-ins and measuring can disappoint and frustrate you – opt instead for a weekly check on how you're doing

We all need a goal to focus our mind on getting what we want out of life, and losing weight is no exception. But how do you stay focused and motivated without getting so fixated on your diet that it takes over your life? It's not easy. The dividing line between focus and obsession is a fine one.

'It's difficult,' admits Andy Hill, a psychologist at Leeds University Medical School and Chairman for the Association for the Study of Obesity. 'But we can distinguish between rigid and flexible dietary approaches.

'Flexible people have a set of principles that they can bend, if necessary,' Andy continues. 'For example, you may allow yourself a certain calorie intake every day, but you can occasionally flout it without feeling guilty or scrapping your diet completely. However, rigid people maintain tight control over their diet until they break the rules, then they lose control, abandon the diet, overeat and feel bad about themselves. It is this rigid behaviour that is associated with obsession.'

Are you an obsessive person?

Although Andy Hill suggests that people who are obsessive about diet may also take a single-minded approach to other aspects of their life, former overeater Gillian Riley thinks the reality is less clear cut.

'I'm not thrilled with the idea of an obsessive personality,' says Gillian, who writes and runs courses on eating less. 'It implies that you can't change, when you *can*.'

So how do you know if you're rigid or flexible, obsessive or not? You probably have an inkling already. If not, our mini quiz could set you on the road to enlightenment.

ARE YOU OBSESSING ABOUT YOUR DIET?

Answer yes or no to the following questions

1. Do you weigh yourself every day? ☐ NO ☐ YES

2. Is your daily mood determined by whether you have lost or gained weight? ☐ NO ☐ YES

3. Have you lost interest in people or activities that used to play an important part in your life? ☐ NO ☐ YES

4. Does your thinking and daily routine revolve around food? ☐ NO ☐ YES

5. Do you stick to a carefully controlled diet and feel bad or defeated when you break it? ☐ NO ☐ YES

Answering 'Yes' to even one of these questions suggests that your approach to weight loss may be too rigid. To lose weight and keep it off for good, follow our experts' advice.

1 SET ACHIEVABLE GOALS

'Obsessional people tend to be driven by goals that are difficult to meet and tend not to be satisfied by interim goals,' says Andy Hill. Setting a series of achievable targets helps you feel as if you're making real progress and stops you getting down about every small setback.

If you tend to obsess about pounds and ounces, try changing your goals so that they aren't specifically about weight loss – but are focused more on taking control of your health and eating habits. For example, instead of vowing to lose 2lb this week, why not choose to walk one mile each day? Whatever you do, stick at it and don't surrender one goal without replacing it with another.

2 LET GO OF 'I MUST' THINKING

'When you think rigidly in terms of "I have to" and "I must", you trigger a sense of rebellion,' says Gillian Riley. 'You suddenly find yourself thinking: "I'm not allowed to eat this packet of biscuits but I'm going to do it anyway." Once you recognise how this kind of thinking is controlling your life, you can break out of it.'

3 EAT TO NURTURE YOURSELF

Starving yourself will not make you lose weight but it could make you sick and unhappy. Instead, start to see food as your friend, an essential and enjoyable part of life that fuels your body, mind and emotions. Eat a varied diet, where nothing is forbidden and make sure you have at least three meals a day. Look after your body – believe that you are worth buying, preparing and eating quality food for.

Aim to learn more about the properties and nutritional value of different foods rather than just concentrating on their calorie and fat content. Abandon out-dated dieting worries such as 'avocados make you fat' – instead relish their delicious creamy flesh that's packed with nutrients that fight heart disease, stroke and cancer.

4 BUILD YOUR SELF-ESTEEM

'A person with low self-esteem will be more attached to pleasing others, which can contribute to obsession,' says Gillian Riley. But self-esteem doesn't mean looking in your mirror and thinking, 'Wow – what a babe', or thriving on compliments from others. 'That isn't really self-esteem at all,' she says.

'Genuine self-esteem is what comes from honouring and valuing yourself – making your own choices, doing what you set out to do, having a sense of purpose and keeping your promises to yourself,' says Gillian Riley.

Gillian Riley's advice is to lay aside the issue of weight loss and focus instead on eating sensibly because you owe it to yourself. 'You can get excited by self-esteem improvement long before you've lost any weight,' says Gillian Riley. 'And the feel-good factor remains long after your diet has ended.'

5 STOKE UP YOUR SOCIAL LIFE

Despite the fact that it may sometimes feel like the most important thing in your life, losing weight is just one part of the happiness package.

'A large component of feeling good about yourself comes from your social life,' says Andy Hill. 'One of the problems with being obsessive about weight loss is that you tend to focus inward and neglect your social life. So, it's vital to balance your weight loss goal with your friendships and other social activities.

'Ask yourself, is it more important to be 3st lighter in one year's time but be left with few friends or outside interests, or to be 1st lighter with a wonderful, busy social life?' The idea is not just to maintain friendships but to extend them by joining clubs, activities and courses.

6 KEEP MUM

Telling other people that you're on a diet only piles on the pressure to succeed and may increase your sense of rebellion. 'It's nice to have your mother, sister or best friend to support you,' says Gillian Riley. 'But even with the best intentions, other people's interest can feel like pressure and may even come across to you as criticism.'

Whatever you achieve should be to meet yours – and not other people's – expectations. Keeping private about what you're doing allows you to stay in control of the issue and ensures you feel free to make your own choices. 'Making your own choice fundamentally changes everything when it comes to fitness and dieting,' says Gillian Riley. 'You have no need to rebel against not being allowed to do or eat something. You just do what is right for you and that itself is life changing.'

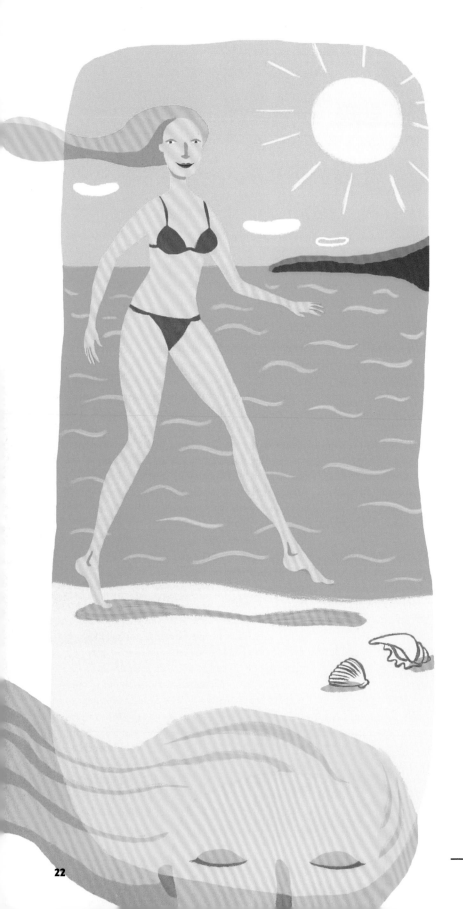

6 secrets of success to get into a slimming frame of mind

Think *yourself* slim

I f you've tried to lose weight and failed, or you find it hard to commit permanently to a healthier way of eating, perhaps you're not using your head. Many health and diet experts agree that slimming starts with a mental approach. In other words, change the way you think and you can change the way you look and feel.

Jane Ogden, a health psychologist at Kings College London, says, 'I've found that the people who lose weight and keep it off are those who believe they can be thin and do something about it. Being slim almost becomes a self-fulfilling prophecy.'

'It's very simple,' agrees Pete Cohen, sports psychologist and founder of the motivational slimming programme, Lighten Up. 'In life, you get what you focus on. Most people focus on what's wrong, what's missing and what they haven't got and they wonder why things don't improve. It's the same with people who want to lose weight,' he claims. 'They focus on what they don't want – the extra weight. But any winner will tell you that the secret of success is to focus on what you *do* want.'

Making your mind work for you

So, how do you make that mental shift? One of the most powerful life-changing tools you can use is visualisation, specifically goal-directed visualisation. Visualisation involves using mental imagery and your senses to encourage relaxation and healing, or to enhance your wellbeing. Goal-directed visualisation simply means you set yourself a goal to focus on; for example, seeing yourself wearing a bikini in six months' time. It's now scientifically proven that your thoughts trigger direct chemical responses in your body, so if you think slim, you make the changes needed to get slim. The theory is that regularly visualising a specific goal means your subconscious mind will direct you towards making that goal a reality in a completely natural and gradual way.

'It's amazing how the brain can generate images of what is possible,' says Pete Cohen. 'Because we tend to think in pictures, you don't need special skills to imagine yourself slimmer in three months' time. Your brain can show you exactly how you'll look. And if you believe that can be you, like a method actor you start to live the part of a slim person and that is who you become.'

The secrets of success

Visualisation is something we can all do. If you close your eyes and picture your last holiday, you're visualising it. However there are certain guidelines that can help you get the most from your imagery:

1 Decide what you want

Do you want to lose weight? Look better? Feel better? Stay healthy? Play football with your kids? Only you know what it is you want, so be specific about your goal. Keep your imagery positive – don't think about losing weight or food, focus on results.

2 Practise until you achieve your goal

Imprint the image so firmly in your subconscious that your mind thinks it's real. 'But try not to spend hours doing it,' says Pete Cohen. 'Just establish an image in your mind and take that image with you wherever you go.' To begin with, however, you may find it easier to focus if you relax in a quiet place and visualise for five to 10 minutes twice a day.

3 Believe and you will achieve

'If you can picture something you believe in it becomes more attainable because you can convince yourself that it's already true,' says Jane Ogden. You have to believe in your goal and your ability to achieve it. For example, you may not believe that you can be a supermodel so you'd never make that your goal, but if you know you could look amazing in the red dress you saw at lunchtime, you'll take steps to slim down to fit into it.

How to visualise yourself slimmer

It's usually best to create your own imagery, as only you know what you want and what works best for you, but the following exercise from Pete Cohen is an easy example of how to use imagery successfully. You may think you have no creative imagination but everyone can picture their own front door. So see if this works for you...

Stand up while you practise

Picture your front door. Familiarise your mind with its size, colour, sturdiness, style and details. Now imagine that standing on the other side of the door is you in three months' time looking slimmer, fitter and healthier.

Open the door in your mind. First of all see yourself from behind. It doesn't matter if you see yourself clearly as long as you know it's you. Most people have no idea what their rear view really looks like so it should be easy to imagine a slim back view. Notice the difference in the clothes you are wearing. Are they your present clothes, only too big? Are you wearing the jeans that haven't fitted you since the Millennium or are you wearing something new? Be specific and detailed. Now turn yourself around so you can see your profile. Notice your complexion, your improved muscle tone, your smile. Next see yourself from the front. Look at how your top accentuates your waist or how those slim-fitting trousers make your legs look slender. If you look well, feel happy and are comfortable with how you look front and back, turn yourself around again so that you have completed a full 360° turn. Now take a step forward so that you 'step into' your image as if you were trying on a new skin.

Alternatively...

● Think of your last holiday – recall the details, sounds and smells and remember how you spent your time. Now look ahead to your next holiday and bring all the detail from the past into the present, only put yourself in the picture looking the way you want to look, feeling the way you want to feel and doing what you want to do.

● Think of a forthcoming event: a birthday party, a wedding or your school reunion. Put yourself in the frame looking slim and feeling happy, see yourself dancing and hear the compliments from friends and relatives.

● Think of what you'd really like to do: play tennis, go swimming, join a salsa class. Forget how you look now, create a new reality looking and feeling gorgeous, and enjoying your life.

● Use affirmations – positive phrases which start with the words 'I am...'. For example, 'I am attractive', 'I am going to be slim', 'I am going to wear that bikini in Turkey'. You see, you can do it!

4 Your destiny is in the detail

Formulate a scene that you want to create. Inject feeling and detail into your visualisation and use all your senses to make your imagery come alive. If you imagine yourself on a beach in a bikini, feel the sun on your skin, smell the sun cream, hear the lapping waves and taste the salt on your lips as if it were real.

5 Set short-term goals

'In my research the people who kept weight off focused on a series of realistic short-term goals because they were more achievable and so more rewarding,' says Jane Ogden. Setting yourself an unattainable goal or one that takes too long to reach only causes stress. So, imagine your goal within a certain timescale, of, say, three or six months. Make your visualisations clear and accurate. What season will it be three months or six months from now? Be realistic about whether you can achieve your goal in that timescale.

6 Talk nicely to yourself

'How you talk to yourself determines how well you coach yourself,' says Pete Cohen. You need to develop a positive internal dialogue. Telling yourself, 'I'm fat, I'm ugly, I never see things through' becomes a self-fulfilling prophecy, so stop saying it. 'You need to replace the bad image with a more positive one,' says Pete Cohen. 'It's about habit breaking. The only way to get rid of a bad habit for good is to replace it with something better.' So tell yourself you are attractive, you are in control and you will succeed.

FEATURE: MARIA MCCARTHY. PHOTOGRAPHY: JON SNEDDON. STYLING: MARIA ZOKAS. HAIR AND MAKE UP: SARAH JANE GREEN AT TERESA FAIRMINER.

3 Must-have tactics for blitzing pounds

HAVE YOU GOT SLIMMING SUSSED?

When you're on a diet it's easy to become fixated on the number of calories or fat grams you're eating and how much exercise you're taking – and to forget everything else. But in order to slim successfully, understanding what you physically need to do to lose weight is only part of the picture. More recently, studies have shown that the women who stick with their exercise and diet programme and manage to keep off the weight long term are the ones who genuinely believe that they will succeed, and who have a positive sense of themselves in the world they live in. Do you fit into this category? Take our quick quiz to find out whether you have the physical, mental and spiritual elements of your diet well covered – the three slimming must-haves – and, if not, just what you need to do to put it right.

1 MUST-HAVE 1: YOUR PHYSICAL HEALTH

Knowing what you should be eating and how much exercise you need to take is vital if you want to lose weight.

1 How often do you exercise?
a) never b) occasionally c) at least three times a week

2 How much water do you drink a day?
a) I only drink tea, coffee and fizzy drinks b) a couple of glasses c) six to eight glasses

3 How many portions of fruit and vegetables do you eat a day?
a) none b) two c) five or more

4 Would you rather have a Mars bar or five pieces of fruit?
a) The Mars bar b) it would depend on how I was feeling c) the fruit

5 When you read a food label do you look at the calorie content only, or do you take into account the fat content, additives etc?
a) I only look at calories b) I look at all the info if I have time c) I always read the whole food label

6 Do you let yourself believe that eating kids' leftovers or food from other people's plates 'doesn't count'?
a) yes b) sometimes c) never

7 Do you go on faddy diets, such as the cabbage soup diet?
a) yes b) sometimes c) never

8 Do you always take the lift instead of the stairs?
a) yes b) sometimes c) no, walking is better exercise

9 How much sleep do you get?
a) less than seven hours a night
b) less than eight hours a night
c) at least eight hours a night

10 Do you eat breakfast?
a) never b) if I have time c) every day

HOW DID YOU DO?

A = 1   B = 3   C = 5
High=25-17, medium=16-10, low=under 10

HIGH
You're clued up about following a healthy diet and exercise plan. Knowing that you're doing something to help you slim keeps you positive, even if you've got lots of weight to lose.
MEDIUM
You could be taking more care of yourself. Rather than exercising when the mood takes you, or just cooking the odd low-fat meal, make a decision to live healthily and stick to it – once you start to lose weight you won't want to undo your hard work.
LOW
If you want to be slim, you have to make practical changes to your life. Start small – go for a walk in your lunch break and snack on fruit instead of crisps, for example, then add in more healthy habits. Try any of the diets in this book or experiment with our low-fat recipes.

2 MUST-HAVE 2: YOUR MENTAL HEALTH

When it comes to slimming, a positive mental attitude is vital. If you believe you really can lose weight you're far more likely to succeed than if you start a diet believing it's destined to fail.

1 How often do you talk about your weight?
a) I talk about little else b) a lot of the time
c) I try not to dwell on it

2 Do you feel envious of slim celebrities?
a) yes, I constantly wish I looked like them
b) sometimes c) I prefer more achievable role models

3 Do you tell yourself being overweight is 'in your genes'?
a) yes – my mum's large so I am too b) sometimes
c) never – I'm the only one in charge of my weight

4 What's your attitude to exercise?
a) I hate it b) I enjoy it once I get going c) I enjoy it

5 How do you feel if you lose 1lb?
a) terrified I'll put it back on b) overjoyed – definitely time for a celebration c) quietly pleased, but ready to tackle the next pound

6 Do you have people you can share your feelings with?
a) no, because no one understands what I'm going through b) I prefer to cope alone c) yes, I feel better when I discuss things with a few trusted friends

7 If you overeat, do you feel guilty that you've blown your diet?
a) I torture myself b) it's horrible, but I don't dwell on it
c) I'm relaxed about it and just get back on track the next day

8 Do you talk negatively about your weight?
a) yes, constantly b) sometimes c) no, never

9 Do you break your weight loss down into specific goals?
a) no, I want to be a size 10 and I won't be happy until I've got there b) yes, if I'm having an off day c) yes, I reward myself with a non-food treat for every ½st lost

10 Do you worry that you'll be overweight forever?
a) Yes, and it terrifies me b) the thought does cross my mind c) no, I'm confident I'll get to my target weight

HOW DID YOU DO?

A = 1   B = 3   C = 5
High=50-35, medium=34-20, low=under 20

HIGH
You've got an excellent mental attitude and this will help you slim. Don't become 'all talk and no action' though. Turn your positive attitude into actions by making lists of different exercises to try, and experiment with new low-fat recipes.

MEDIUM
You've got room for improvement. Get support from family and repeat a mantra, like 'I can be slim', to help you believe you can lose weight.

LOW
It's hard to slim if you think negatively about yourself and your body, so stop it – no more wailing to your boyfriend that your bum looks big, for example. After a few weeks you'll notice a difference and feel more positive, and will have made a step towards breaking out of unhelpful mental patterns.

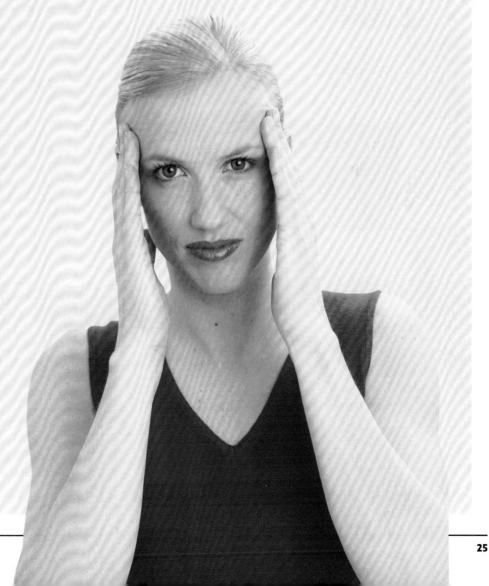

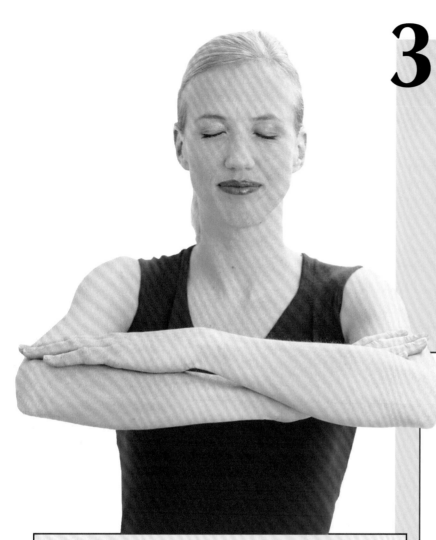

3 MUST-HAVE 3: YOUR SPIRITUAL HEALTH

Being spiritually balanced is all to do with feeling OK about yourself and your life as a whole, and accepting any imperfections you have.

1 Do you like yourself?
a) no b) most of the time c) yes

2 Are you kind to other people?
a) not particularly – I don't think they'd put themselves out for me b) I try to be c) yes, my motto is 'do as you would be done by' and I try to live by it

3 Do you feel you have to shut yourself away from the rest of the world until you've lost weight?
a) yes, I can't bear the thought of being judged by other people b) if I have a 'fat day' I don't really feel like going out c) no, life is what's happening around me now, not what's going to happen when I'm slim

4 When planning your week, where do you come in your list of priorities?
a) generally bottom of the list b) about midway down c) wherever I come, I always make sure I have some time for myself

5 Do you feel grateful for the good things in your life?
a) what good things? b) sometimes c) yes, always

HOW DID YOU DO?

A = 1   B = 3   C = 5
High=25-17, medium=16-10, low=under 10

HIGH
Your approach to life has a strong spiritual basis. That doesn't necessarily mean that you're religious, but more that you've got a generous, accepting attitude towards yourself and other people. That helps you value yourself, regardless of your weight – and in turn makes you more likely to succeed in your weight loss goals.

MEDIUM
You have quite good spiritual awareness, but you could build on it by thinking about yourself more and by not putting off life because of your weight. To give yourself more opportunity to evaulate and consider, you might like to try yoga and meditation. Meditation is particularly effective for helping you pull back from everyday worries and keeping you relaxed – useful from a dieting point of view if you overeat when you're stressed.

LOW
If you find it hard to like yourself, think about how to build your self-esteem. Make a 'gratitude list' of all the things you've got to be grateful for in life and think about them when you feel you might be getting obsessed about your weight. Giving yourself non-food treats will also help you think of yourself as a worthwhile person who deserves care. If you have time, doing voluntary work can help you take a spiritual approach to life – as well as keeping your mind off food.

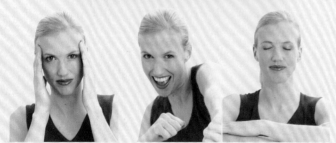

Getting the 3 must-haves in place

If this quiz has shown you that you're making the right choices in one or two parts of your life – but not all three – don't panic. All you need to do is make some simple adjustments to get the other ones up to speed. But once all three areas of your life – the physical, mental and spiritual – are on track, your diet will be too. And that's a promise we can guarantee!

HOW HEALTHY IS YOUR DIET?

7 questions to put yourself to the test

Every slimmer knows how to count calories, but how much do you really know about the foods you should be eating to lose weight healthily? To find out how high you score in nutrition know-how, try our easy healthy-eating QUIZ…

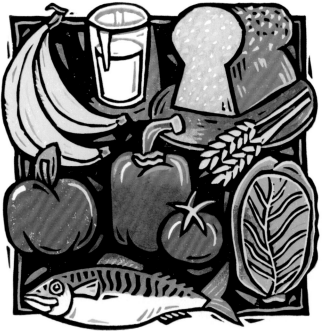

1 The following is a list of the ingredients in a typical muesli bar: sugar, rolled oats, dextrose, wheat flakes, rice, fructose, corn syrup, partially hydrogenated peanut oil, skimmed milk powder, almonds, malt, sorbitol and flavouring. How many of these ingredients are actually different types of sugar?

A One ☐   B Three ☐   C Five ☐   D Six ☐

2 You've heard of the concept of 'good' fats and 'bad' fats. But which of the types of fats listed below should you avoid the most?
A Saturated fat ☐
B Hydrogenated fat (also known as trans fat) ☐
C Monounsaturated fat ☐
D Polyunsaturated fat ☐

3 How much fat should you include in your diet if you want to lose weight and stay healthy?
A As little as possible ☐
B Less than 20% of your total daily calorie intake ☐
C 25 to 30% of your total daily calorie intake ☐
D 30 to 35% of your total daily calorie intake ☐

4 Women need a recommended 14.8mg iron per day. Can you put the following foods in order according to which contains the most iron?
A One egg ☐
B 75g/3oz lean beef ☐
C 100g/3½oz quinoa ☐
D 1tbsp blackstrap molasses ☐

5 Which of the following statements about protein are correct?
A Protein makes you feel fuller for longer ☐
B Protein doesn't just come from animal products, vegetarians can get a good supply of protein from plant sources ☐
C The recommended protein intake for women is 45g per day ☐
D Peanuts and Cheddar cheese contain almost the same amount of protein, gram for gram ☐

6 Most people need to eat more fibre, say the experts, as the average consumption of around 12g per day is well below the daily recommendation of 18g. So which of the following breakfast cereals has the most fibre per serving?
A Cornflakes ☐
B Branflakes ☐
C Muesli ☐
D Porridge ☐

7 According to Government recommendations, women need at least 700mg of calcium a day to keep their bones healthy – and women who are on a weight-loss plan tend to miss out on the full amount they need. Which of the following comes closest to providing you with your daily requirement of calcium?
A 100g/3½oz tofu ☐
B 450ml/16floz of skimmed milk ☐
C 50g bar of milk chocolate ☐
D 100g/3½oz Cheddar cheese ☐

HOW DID YOU SCORE?

Give yourself a point for each correct answer

1D Sugar, dextrose, fructose, corn syrup, malt and sorbitol are all types of sugars. So even if you don't add sugar to tea or coffee, you could still be getting more than the recommended amount (10% of your total calorie intake) thanks to the hidden sugars in most processed foods – even in so-called 'healthy' foods such as muesli bars. Always check the food labels on any pre-prepared, processed foods you buy, especially low-fat foods, which are notoriously packed full of added sugars. Look out for ingredients that end in 'ose', such as sucrose, glucose, dextrose, fructose, galactose, lactose, polydextrose and maltodextrose – these are all just fancy words for plain old sugar. Other sneaky sugars include honey, corn and fruit syrups, fruit juice concentrates, plus ingredients that sound like artificial sweeteners (but are actually naturally derived sugars) such as mannitol, xylitol and sorbitol.

2B Hydrogenation is a chemical process that turns unsaturated fats into saturated fats – in other words, it turns them from oils into fats that are solid at room temperature. Experts claim that these fats are particularly bad for you because, as they're man-made, the human body can't digest them properly. As a result, they've been linked with many health problems, most notably heart disease. You'll find them in bakery foods such as cakes and biscuits, plus some margarines, salad creams, crisps and breads. Current Government guidelines state that no more than 2% of your daily calories should come from hydrogenated fats, so look out for them on food labels. Meanwhile, if your answer was (a), saturated fat, you weren't too far off the mark. Saturated fats have been linked with high cholesterol problems, so it's a good idea to limit your intake of these, too (no more than 10% of total calorie intake). They're mostly found in meat and full-fat dairy products.

3C Over the years, slimmers have been conditioned to think that the less fat you eat, the more weight you'll lose. This is true to a broad extent, but cutting fat out of your diet completely is not a healthy option. Without a certain amount of fat in your diet you could develop health problems ranging from dry skin and hair, to more serious conditions such as depression and arthritis. What's more, many experts now claim that fat helps to make you feel full – so if you include some fat in your diet, you may actually eat fewer calories overall. Most dieticians recommend that around 25-30% of your total calories should come from fat if you want to lose weight healthily – that's 42g to 50g if you're eating 1,500 calories a day. If you've already achieved your target weight, aim for 33% (55g).

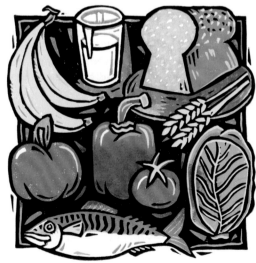

FEATURE: CHRISTINE MORGAN. ILLUSTRATIONS: ILLUSTRATION WORKS

Lose weight the healthy way

4C, D, B, A If you're wondering what quinoa is, it's a grain from South America that's well worth getting to know as it's such a rich source of iron (it also contains lots of vitamin B1 plus protein, calcium, vitamin B2 and niacin). Just 100g/3½oz of quinoa contains 8mg iron – that's over half your daily requirement. Buy it from health food shops and use it instead of rice or couscous. Blackstrap molasses – a thick, black syrup, is also available from health food shops and contains 3.5mg iron per tablespoon, but be careful as it's high in sugar. Surprisingly, 75g/3oz lean beef only gives you 2.5g iron, and an egg contains just 1mg. But why should you be concerned about getting more iron? Well, it's a fact that most women don't get enough, especially those who are on a calorie-controlled diet. Experts claim we need to eat 2,500 to 3,000 calories a day to get the amount of iron we need from a typical diet, so if you're getting 1,500 calories or less, your chances of having an iron deficiency are pretty high. And if you're not getting enough iron you can suffer from anaemia, the classic signs of which are constant tiredness and light-headedness.

5 ALL When you're on a calorie-controlled diet, eating some protein at every meal will help to control your appetite because it takes longer to digest than carbohydrates, so you won't feel hungry so soon afterwards. And yes, there are many good sources of protein from both animal and plant sources – for instance, beef, turkey, prawns and red kidney beans all have over 20g protein per 100g. Peanuts and Cheddar cheese contain 25.6g and 25.5g per 100g, respectively. Some experts claim that you should aim to get more of your protein from plant sources than animal products, as meat and dairy foods tend to contain higher levels of saturated fat.

6B As more evidence is uncovered about high-fibre diets reducing the risk of some cancers and heart disease, it's worth making sure you're getting the recommended amount. Slimmers in particular can also benefit from eating more fibre, as high-fibre foods fill you up with relatively few calories. Branflakes contain 3.9g fibre per 30g, with the humble cornflake lagging behind miserably with 0.3g for the same size serving. A bowl of porridge contains around 1.6g fibre, while muesli has 2g. Even better than all these are bran strand cereals such as All Bran, which contain just under 10g fibre per 40g serving.

7D Dairy products are by far the best source of calcium – 100g of Cheddar cheese contains a whopping 720mg. But you wouldn't want to eat that much cheese in a day as it contains over 400 calories and more than 30g fat, the majority of which is saturated. Low-fat cheeses are a healthier option, but even these are relatively high in fat. The better choice is 450ml/16floz skimmed milk, which contains a reasonable 540mg calcium and only 158 calories, plus just under a gram of fat. If, on the other hand, you're lactose intolerant or you don't eat dairy foods, tofu is similarly rich in calcium with 510mg per 100g. The bar of chocolate, by the way, contains just 100mg calcium – so there goes that excuse. Other great sources of calcium include green leafy vegetables, sesame seeds, sardines, seaweed and salmon (canned with bones).

WHAT YOUR SCORE MEANS

6-7 POINTS Well done. Keep up the good work – it will pay huge dividends in terms of your health and your weight for years to come.

4-5 POINTS Pretty good. Your nutrition know-how is reasonably healthy and hopefully this shows in your food choices.

3 POINTS OR LESS You've got a lot to learn about nutrition – but don't worry. Read through the various healthy eating articles in this book to help you make the right food choices.

DIETS

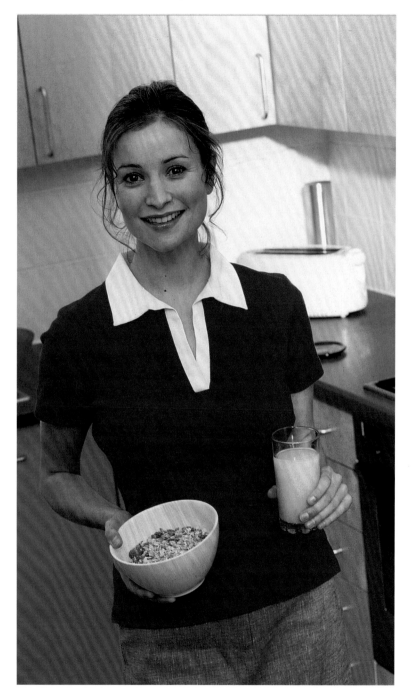

H as your diet hit a plateau? Or perhaps you want to kick-start a new plan into action? This dead easy three-day programme will have you burning fat and calories faster than you can say 'reduced-fat Cheddar'. So what are you waiting for? Give it a go right now…

Here's what to do

● Decide whether you want to count calories or fat grams. We've included two plans because we know that some of you are more comfortable counting calories and others are happier monitoring your fat intake. We've covered the bases by giving vegetarian options for each meal (flagged with a V). All recipes serve one.
● Choose a different breakfast, light meal and main meal each day to ensure you get a wide variety of nutrients. But don't switch between the

calorie and fat plans.
● Every day have 275ml/¹/₂pt skimmed milk for tea and coffee or to drink on its own. This is on top of any milk that appears in the meals. If you prefer, you may have two small pots of diet yoghurt instead. Milk and yoghurt are sources of calcium – essential for healthy bones – so don't miss out on this allowance.
● You may drink unlimited amounts of water, black tea and coffee, herbal teas, Bovril, Marmite and diet or low-calorie soft drinks.
● As well as your three meals you may also have unlimited amounts of most vegetables, see the 'Free' vegetables box.
● Where a fruit option is included with a meal you may save it to eat separately as a snack.
● **Note:** All teaspoon (tsp) and tablespoon (tbsp) measurements should be level.

Whether you're just starting your diet or you've hit a plateau, use this no-nonsense, three-day eating plan to get you on track and lose up to 3lb in three days

The **kick-start** diet

Breakfasts

Counting calories: breakfasts (250 calories)

Bacon and tomato ciabatta roll
Slice a 50g/2oz ciabatta bread roll and fill with 2 lean rashers back bacon, grilled, 1 tomato, sliced, and 1tbsp tomato ketchup or brown sauce.

Poached egg with tomato (V)
Toast 50g/2oz crusty French bread and top with 1 medium egg, poached, plus 1 tomato, grilled.

Greek fruit salad (V)
Chop 1 orange and 1 small banana and mix with 50g/2oz canteloupe melon. Top with 1tbsp unsweetened muesli, 2tbsp fat-free Greek yoghurt and 1tsp runny honey.

Fruit brioche (V)
Place a brioche roll, halved, on a grill pan and top with 50g/2oz defrosted summer fruit mixture (available from supermarkets). Drizzle 1tsp runny honey over the top and place under a medium grill until warm.

Apricot muesli (V)
Mix 40g/1½oz unsweetened muesli with 3 dried apricots and 150ml/¼pt skimmed milk.

Toast and honey with fruit (V)
Spread 2 medium slices wholemeal toast with 2tsp low-fat spread and 2tsp honey. Plus 1 kiwi fruit.

Counting fat grams: breakfasts (5g fat)

Mushrooms, bacon and toast
Grill 5 rashers unsmoked rindless bacon and serve with 1 thick slice wholemeal toast topped with 100g/3½oz chestnut mushrooms, fried in 2tsp low-fat spread.

Toasted muffin with strawberries (V)
Halve and toast 1 teacake and spread with 1tsp low-fat spread and 2tsp reduced-sugar jam. Plus strawberries.

Cereal and toast (V)
30g low-fat cereal with 150ml/¼pt skimmed milk, plus 1 thick slice wholemeal toast with 2tsp low-fat spread.

Toasted muffin with cream cheese (V)
Halve and toast 1 English wholemeal muffin. Spread with 25g/1oz reduced-fat cream cheese.

Ham and mustard bagel with fruit
1 wholemeal bagel filled with 2tsp low-fat spread, a scraping of mustard and 50g/2oz wafer thin ham. Plus 1 kiwi fruit.

Toasted muffin and beans with yoghurt and apple (V)
Toast 1 wholemeal English muffin, spread with 2tsp low-fat spread and top with 150g/5oz baked beans, heated. Plus 100g pot low-fat yoghurt and apple.

'Free' vegetables
You may eat unlimited amounts of the following vegetables: artichokes, asparagus, aubergines, bean sprouts, broccoli, Brussels sprouts, cabbage, carrots, cauliflower, celery, chicory, courgettes, cucumber, fennel, garlic, gherkins, green beans, leeks, lettuce, mangetout, marrow, mushrooms, onions, peppers, pumpkins, radish, spinach, spring greens, swede, tomatoes, turnip and watercress.

How much weight will I lose?
Follow this diet and you can expect to lose around 3lb in three days. Each daily menu, including the milk allowance, provides 1,000 calories or 28g fat. This plan is designed to get your healthy eating off to a good start or to help you shift a few stubborn pounds. The calorie/fat allowance is very low, so don't follow it for any longer than three days, as you'll be losing muscle as well as fat, which isn't good for your health.
   Once your three days are up, switch to one of the other diets in this Chapter.

Light meals

Counting calories: light meals (300 calories)

Tuna sandwich and crisps
Fill 2 medium slices wholemeal bread with 50g/2oz tuna, drained of brine, and unlimited 'free' salad. Plus 25g packet low-fat crisps.

Ploughman's with yoghurt (V)
Serve 2 medium slices wholemeal bread with 25g/1oz reduced-fat Cheddar cheese, 2tsp pickle and unlimited 'free' salad. Plus 125g pot diet yoghurt.

Soup with fromage frais
Heat 295g can Weight Watchers from Heinz Minestrone Soup and serve with 50g/2oz wholemeal roll. Plus 1 small banana and 100g pot diet fromage frais.

Baked potato (V)
Bake a 200g/7oz potato (raw weight), and top with 65g/2½oz reduced-fat houmous.

Chicken Waldorf pitta
Combine 40g/1½oz skinless chicken (cooked weight); 1 apple, chopped; 1tsp lemon juice; 2 sticks celery, chopped; ½ small onion, chopped; and 1tsp reduced-calorie mayo and use to fill 75g/3oz wholemeal pitta bread. Plus unlimited 'free' salad.

Bagel with fruit (V)
Fill 1 wholemeal bagel with 50g/2oz reduced-fat soft cheese and unlimited 'free' salad. Plus 1 kiwi fruit.

Light meals (continued)

Bean and coleslaw pitta (V)
Fill 1 wholemeal pitta bread with 50g/2oz red kidney beans, canned and drained, 115g/4oz reduced-calorie coleslaw and unlimited 'free' salad.

Burger in a bun with banana and yoghurt
Grill a 50g/2oz low-fat burger and serve in a soft white roll with sliced tomato, lettuce and chopped onion. Follow with 1 small pot plain low-fat yoghurt and 1 small banana.

Cheese jacket potato with sorbet cone (V)
Bake a 200g/7oz potato (raw weight), fill with 40g/1½oz reduced-fat Cheddar cheese, grated, and spring onions, sliced. Serve with unlimited 'free' vegetables. Follow with 100g/3½oz raspberry sorbet in an ice cream cone.

Ham salad roll
Spread 1 large wholemeal roll with 2tsp low-fat spread and fill with 50g/2oz lean ham and unlimited 'free' salad.

Vegetable stir-fry with yoghurt (V)
Boil 50g/2oz brown rice (raw weight). Heat 1tsp vegetable oil in a nonstick pan and stir-fry a section of 'free' vegetables, such as: bean sprouts, onions, peppers, carrots, broccoli and mangetout, until cooked. Serve with the rice and 1tbsp soy sauce. Plus 1 small pot low-fat bio fruit yoghurt.

Jacket potato with tuna and sweetcorn
Bake a 200g/7oz potato (raw weight). Mix together 1tbsp sweetcorn, 150g/5oz tuna, drained of brine, and 2tbsp reduced-calorie mayonnaise and use to fill the potato. Serve with unlimited 'free' salad.

Roast pork with satsuma
Serve 75g/3oz lean roast pork, 75g/3oz roast potatoes, and 2tbsp unsweetened apple sauce with unlimited 'free' vegetables and 4tbsp fat-free gravy. Plus 1 satsuma.

Bruschetta and salad (V)
Place 1 red pepper, deseeded and thickly sliced; 2 plum tomatoes, halved; 1 courgette, sliced; and 2 shallots, peeled and halved, on a baking tray and brush with 1tsp olive oil. Sprinkle with fresh basil, chopped, and black pepper. Place in a hot oven for 20 minutes. Warm a 50g/2oz slice of ciabatta bread and spread with 2tsp pesto sauce. Pile on the roasted vegetables and juices. Serve with unlimited 'free' salad.

Egg florentine (V)
Lightly steam 200g/7oz spinach until the leaves wilt, then place in an ovenproof dish. At the same time poach 1 medium egg, and carefully place on top of the spinach. Sprinkle with 25g/1oz reduced-fat Cheddar cheese, grated. Grill until melted and serve with 50g/2oz French bread.

Fish and chips with fromage frais
Grill 1 cod fishcake and serve with 115g/4oz low-fat oven chips, 75g/3oz garden peas and 1tbsp tomato ketchup. Plus 100g pot diet fromage frais.

Pasta and tomato sauce with apple (V)
Cook 50g/2oz wholewheat pasta and combine with ½ x 475g jar of light pasta sauce. Sprinkle with 2tbsp Parmesan cheese, grated, and serve with unlimited 'free' vegetables. Plus 1 apple.

Ready meal with fromage frais
300 calorie ready meal, served with unlimited 'free' vegetables. Plus 100g pot diet fromage frais.

Prawn and red pesto swirls
Cook 40g/1½oz pasta swirls. Drain and toss in 1½tbsp red pesto sauce. Add 40g/1½oz prawns, and 50g/1oz button mushrooms – lightly dry-fried in a nonstick pan to soften – and toss to coat them in the pesto. Season with pepper, 1tbsp chopped fresh coriander and the zest of 1 lemon. Serve warm with unlimited 'free' vegetables.

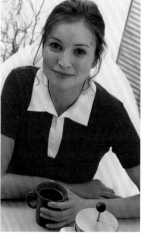

Bacon-wrapped chicken and soft cheese
Stuff a 150g/5oz skinless, boneless chicken breast (raw weight) with 25g/1oz reduced-fat cream cheese and wrap with 25g/1oz streaky bacon. Bake in a medium oven for at least 20 minutes and serve with unlimited 'free' vegetables.

'American hot' pizza and salad (V)
Preheat the oven to 180°C/350°F/gas mark 4. Top a medium pizza base with 200g can chopped tomatoes, drained; mushrooms, sliced; spring onions, sliced; ½ red pepper, deseeded and sliced; 1tsp fresh chilli, finely chopped; and 25g/1oz reduced-fat Cheddar cheese, grated. Bake for 10 minutes and serve with unlimited 'free' salad.

Bean chilli with ice cream (V)
Mix a 200g can chopped tomatoes and herbs with 200g can mixed bean salad, ½tsp chilli powder, 1 crushed garlic clove and pepper. Heat through thoroughly then sprinkle with 25g/1oz reduced-fat Cheddar cheese, grated, and serve with 75g/3oz brown rice (raw weight), boiled. Plus 50g/2oz low-calorie vanilla ice cream.

Poached salmon
Serve 150g/5oz salmon fillet, poached, with 4 small new potatoes. Plus unlimited 'free' vegetables.

Ready meal with fruit (V)
15g fat ready meal, served with unlimited 'free' vegetables. Plus 1 orange.

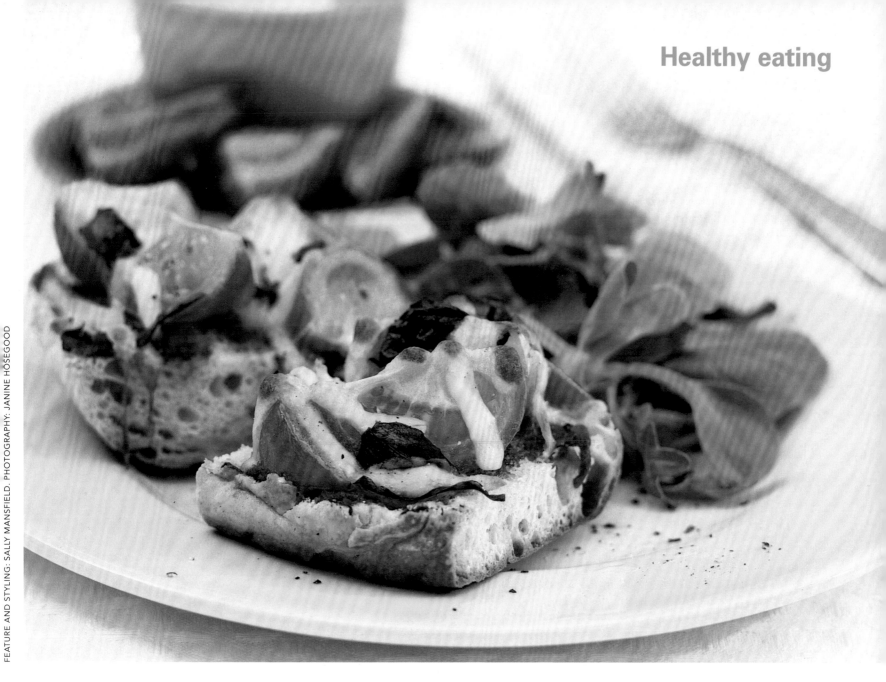

FEATURE AND STYLING: SALLY MANSFIELD. PHOTOGRAPHY: JANINE HÖSEGOOD

Your *energy* diet

Try our uplifting energy diet. It's packed with nutrients and tasty food – start today and be 1st lighter in six weeks!

Our energy-packed diet aims to get you in shape AND have you feeling fit. Within just six weeks you can lose up to 1st, although in the long term, you should aim to shift 1lb to 2lb a week (you might drop more weight when you first start due to loss of water as well as fat). If you regularly shed more than 2lb a week, you'll be losing muscle, too, so keep within your calorie allowance (see below) and don't go below 1,250 calories a day.

Your calorie quota
● **Less than 1st to lose: 1,250 calories a day.**
INCLUDES one 250-cal snack.
● **Between 1st and 3st to lose: 1,250 cals a day,**
INCLUDES two 250-cal snacks.
● **More than 3st to lose: 1,500 cals a day, INCLUDES**
three 250-cal snacks.
■ **Total calories include three meals, daily dairy allowance**
and your snack/s.

What do I do?
● **Pick one breakfast, one light meal, one main meal and your snack/s according to your allowance each day (see above), varying your choices so you don't get bored.**
● **As well as meals (and snacks), have 275ml/ ¹/₂pt skimmed milk each day on its own or for tea and coffee, in addition to any milk that appears in the menus. Or have 2 x 125g pots diet yoghurt, or 150ml/¹/₄pt skimmed milk plus 125g pot diet yoghurt.**
● **You can eat unlimited amounts of the veg listed below – raw or lightly cooked – at all midday and evening meals. Be sure to eat three different portions of veg (count a salad as one) and vary what you eat.**
● **You can drink unlimited amounts of water, very weak tea, coffee, low-calorie or diet squashes and fizzy drinks, Bovril and Marmite.**

Fill up on these 'free' veggies:

Artichoke, asparagus, aubergine, beansprouts, broccoli, Brussels sprouts, cabbage, carrots, cauliflower, celery, chicory, courgettes, cucumber, fennel, garlic, gherkins, green beans, leek, lettuce, mangetout, marrow, mushrooms, onion, pepper, pumpkin, radish, spinach, spring greens, swede, tomatoes, turnip and watercress.

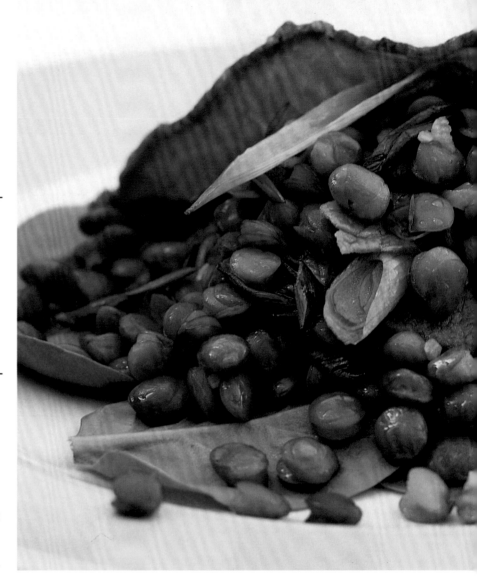

Breakfasts 200 calories

CEREAL AND CARROT JUICE
2 Weetabix with 150ml/¹/₄pt skimmed milk and 150ml/¹/₄pt glass carrot juice.

STRAWBERRY SMOOTHIE
Blend 200g/7oz strawberries with 125g pot diet strawberry yoghurt and 275ml/¹/₂pt skimmed milk.

PINEAPPLE AND KIWI YOGHURT
200g/7oz fresh diced pineapple (or pineapple canned in natural juice), 1 peeled, diced kiwi fruit and 125g pot natural low-fat bio yoghurt.

BANANA CEREAL
3tbsp bran cereal with 150ml/¹/₄pt skimmed milk and 1 small banana.

Light meals 300 calories

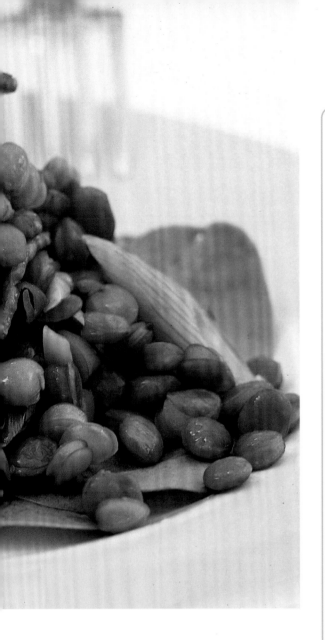

SANDWICH CHOICE

2 medium slices wholemeal bread with 1tsp low-fat spread and your choice of one of the following fillings, plus salad:
- 1/2 small sliced avocado, 1 grilled slice lean back bacon and lettuce leaves.
- 2tbsp low-fat cottage cheese, 75g/3oz tuna in brine.

WARM BACON, LENTIL AND SPINACH SALAD

Heat 2tsp oil in a non-stick pan and gently sauté 2 sliced spring onions, 1 garlic clove, crushed, 2 lean rashers back bacon and 1/2 x 400g can green lentils, drained. Cook for 5 minutes and serve on a bed of baby spinach leaves.

CRUDITÉS AND DIP

Prepare a selection of raw vegetables of your choice for dipping (try celery, carrots, peppers, cucumber, spring onions, cauliflower) plus 5 breadsticks, and serve with 3 1/2tbsp taramasalata, 5tbsp houmous or 4tbsp sour cream and chive dip.

SMOKED TROUT SALAD

75g/3oz cooked smoked trout fillet with 200g/7oz new potatoes plus vegetables.

GARLIC ROAST TOMATOES

Slice 4 fresh plum tomatoes in half and place in an ovenproof dish. Sprinkle with 1tbsp olive oil, 2 crushed garlic cloves, torn basil leaves and freshly ground black pepper. Place in a hot oven for 20 minutes and serve with 40g/1 1/2oz crusty bread.

CRUNCHY FRUIT AND NUT SALAD

Mix together 4 chopped, ready-to-eat dried apricots, 1 small chopped apple, 1 small grated courgette, 1/2 chopped red onion, 1 small grated carrot, 3tbsp reduced-calorie coleslaw, 3 chopped walnut halves and 1tsp fresh chopped parsley.

CHICKEN IN A BUN

Grill 115g/4oz chicken breast fillet and serve up in a small wholemeal bread roll with 1 medium sliced tomato, some crisp lettuce and 1tbsp reduced-calorie mayonnaise.

BRUSCHETTA

Sprinkle 1tsp extra virgin olive oil over 40g/1 1/2oz crusty bread and grill. Top with half a serving roasted veggies (see *Healthy Roasties*, pg. 37).

POACHED EGG ON TOAST

1 poached egg on 1 medium slice wholemeal toast and 150ml/1/4pt orange juice.

TOMATOES ON TOAST

1 medium slice wholemeal toast with 400g can peeled plum tomatoes. 125g pot diet yoghurt.

MUESLI AND MELON

2tbsp unsweetened muesli with 150ml/1/4pt skimmed milk, 200g/7oz melon.

TOAST AND CRANBERRY JUICE

1 medium slice wholemeal toast with 1tsp low-fat spread and 1tsp jam or marmalade. Also have 150ml/1/4pt unsweetened cranberry juice.

BREAKFAST-TO-GO

Choose from 1 hot cross bun with 2tsp low-fat spread; or 1 Jordan's Frusli (any flavour); or Crunchy bar. Plus 150ml/1/4pt unsweetened orange juice.

BEAN SALAD

Mix 1/2 x 400g can mixed beans with 1 grated carrot, 1/2 sliced red onion, 4 sliced cherry tomatoes and 2tbsp fat-free vinaigrette. Serve with 40g/1 1/2oz crusty bread.

BAKED SALMON, RICE AND VEGETABLES

Wrap 115g/4oz skinless salmon fillet in foil and place on a baking tray in a medium oven for 20 minutes. Serve with 50g/2oz rice and some steamed vegetables.

MOZZARELLA MELT AND STRAWBERRIES

Top 40g/1$\frac{1}{2}$oz ciabatta bread with 2tsp pesto sauce, 1 sliced tomato, 40g/1$\frac{1}{2}$oz grated mozzarella and torn basil leaves. Place in a medium oven for 20 minutes. Serve with salad. Follow with 200g/7oz strawberries and 125g pot diet yoghurt.

BANANA CHICKEN STIR-FRY

Heat 1tsp oil in a non-stick pan or wok and cook 1 garlic clove, crushed, and $\frac{1}{2}$in chopped root ginger until soft. Add 115g/4oz lean chicken breast fillet, diced, and cook for about 10 minutes. Mix 5tbsp orange juice with 1tbsp soy sauce, 1tbsp dry sherry and 1tsp cornflour, and add to the pan. Toss a small diced banana in 1tsp lemon juice and add to the pan with $\frac{1}{2}$ small diced avocado. Heat gently for a few minutes. Serve with vegetables.

PORK AND ROASTED VEG

Grill 115g/4oz lean pork loin. Serve with $\frac{1}{2}$ serving roast veg and 200g/7oz new potatoes.

EGG-FRIED VEGETABLE RICE

Heat 2tsp oil in a non-stick pan and gently fry 1 garlic clove, crushed, $\frac{1}{2}$ chopped onion, $\frac{1}{2}$ diced red pepper, a pinch of crushed chilli flakes (or $\frac{1}{2}$tsp chilli powder) and 6 halved button mushrooms, until soft. Remove from pan and put to one side. Add 1 beaten egg to pan and stir on a low heat until cooked. Return vegetables to the pan and add 50g/2oz cooked rice. Heat through.

CAULIFLOWER AND BROCCOLI CHEESE AND POTATOES

Heat 150ml/$\frac{1}{4}$pt skimmed milk in a pan. Mix 1tbsp cornflour with 2tbsp skimmed milk and add to the pan. Heat the milk, stirring all the time, until it thickens. Add 40g/1$\frac{1}{2}$oz grated reduced-fat Cheddar cheese plus 1 bay leaf and freshly-ground black pepper. Place some just-cooked broccoli and cauliflower florets in an oven-proof dish, pour cheese sauce over the top and place under a hot grill for 5 minutes. Serve with 275g/10oz jacket potato.

ENGLISH BREAKFAST

Grill 2 lean rashers back bacon, 1 large reduced-fat pork sausage and 2 halved tomatoes. Serve with 1 poached egg, 1medium slice wholemeal toast and 150ml/$\frac{1}{4}$pt orange juice.

WARM CHICKEN PASTA SALAD

Mix together 50g/2oz pasta shapes, 75g/3oz lean, cooked, diced chicken, 4 sliced cherry tomatoes, $\frac{1}{2}$ diced red onion, 1tsp fresh parsley, and dressing made of 1tsp oil, 1tsp white wine vinegar, 1tsp lemon juice and $\frac{1}{2}$tsp mustard.

HOMEMADE BEEFBURGERS

Mix together 115g/4oz extra-lean minced beef, $\frac{1}{2}$ beaten egg, 2tbsp fresh wholemeal breadcrumbs, $\frac{1}{2}$ grated onion and some freshly ground black pepper. Mould the beef mixture into 2 burger shapes and cook under the grill for 15 minutes, turning after 7 minutes. Serve with 1 small wholemeal bread roll and 1tbsp tomato ketchup.

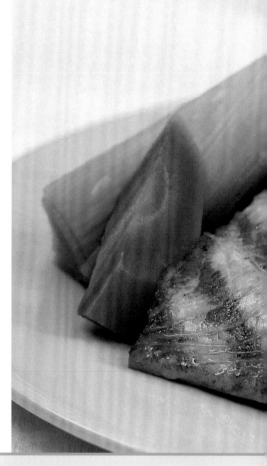

Things to do with veg...

Perk up your vegetable by trying different varieties and new ways of cooking them...

● Stir-fry, roast, grill or add to your favourite dishes – even if they're not in the recipe.

● Be adventurous – try artichokes, celeriac, chicory and okra.

● Munch on raw veg such as peppers, cauliflower, courgette and carrots. They're low-calorie and retain nutrients often lost during the heat of cooking. Add them to your leaf, rice and pasta salads.

● If you can't be bothered to prepare vegetables, don't skip them – spend a little extra and buy them pre-prepared. It's worth it if it means the difference between eating them or not.

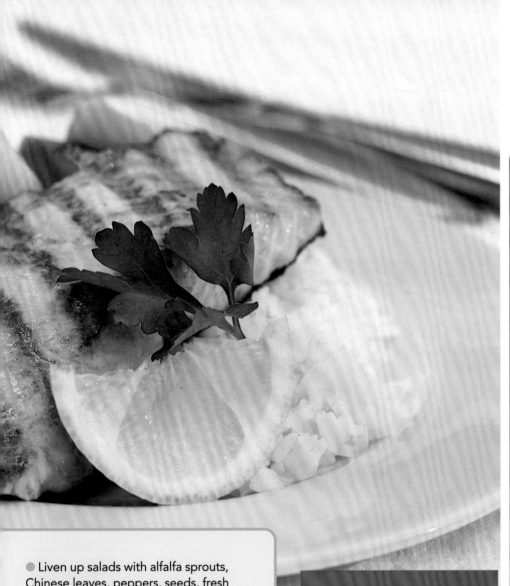

Snacks 250 cals

Choose from these daily 250-calorie extras...

Choose from one, two or three of these snacks:
● Fruit: 1 medium banana, 1 nectarine, 200g/7oz strawberries, 200g/7oz melon.
● Pasta and pesto: cook 50g/2oz pasta and mix with 2tsp pesto sauce and 1tbsp grated Parmesan.
● Mozzarella treat: Arrange 1 large sliced beef tomato on a plate with 40g/1^1/$_2$oz sliced mozzarella cheese. Sprinkle with white wine vinegar and fresh chopped basil. Serve with 1 medium slice wholemeal bread.
● Fruit pot: Place 200g/7oz defrosted summer fruits in a blender with 125g pot diet strawberry yoghurt, 1tsp honey and 275ml/^{1}/$_2$pt skimmed milk. Blend and mix with 3tbsp cereal.
● 4tbsp cereal, 150ml/^{1}/$_4$pt skimmed milk, 150ml/^{1}/$_4$pt glass orange juice, 125g pot diet yoghurt.
● 1 medium slice wholemeal toast spread with 205g can baked beans in tomato sauce.
● 2 medium slices wholemeal bread with 1tsp low-fat spread, 75g/3oz canned tuna in brine, 1 sliced tomato.
● 50g bag mixed peanuts and raisins.
● 40g/1^1/$_2$oz salted, shelled almonds.
● ^{1}/$_2$pt lager, bitter or cider or 125ml glass wine or 1 pub measure of whisky, gin or vodka with a diet mixer plus 30g bag crisps.
● 50g bar chocolate.

You can liven up your veg allowance:
● Salad dressing made from 2tbsp olive oil, 2tsp white wine vinegar, 1tsp lemon juice, ^{1}/$_2$tsp mustard and freshly-ground black pepper.
● 2^1/$_2$tbsp mayonnaise or 5^1/$_2$tbsp reduced-calorie mayo or 5tbsp salad cream or 3tbsp regular French dressing.
● 2^1/$_2$tbsp butter or 2tbsp oil.
● 75g/3oz reduced-fat grated Cheddar cheese or have 50g/2oz grated fresh Parmesan cheese.

● Liven up salads with alfalfa sprouts, Chinese leaves, peppers, seeds, fresh herbs, bean sprouts, grated courgette, grated carrot, spinach or watercress.
● Steam your veg, as this method retains maximum nutrients and flavour. If you do boil them, only just cover them with water and don't over cook them.
● If you have more than 1st to lose you can use your extra calorie allowance to add flavour to your salad and vegetables. Have oils, dressings, butter and cheese, instead.
● Frozen vegetables have the reputation of being inferior to fresh. In fact, they're often more nutritious, as they are usually frozen soon after harvesting, which can retain the nutrients.

Healthy roasties

Using the veggies from your daily allowance, cut into chunks or slices, drizzle over 2tbsp olive oil and coat using your hands, then add garlic cloves and fresh herbs. Roast in a hot oven for 25 minutes until golden brown.
● 250 calories per serving (2tbsp oil) – allowed if you have 1st or more to lose. If not, you can try dry roasting them.

Your 30 minutes

Spend no more than half an hour in the kitchen a day – and shift pounds...

Do you put off starting diets because you think they're too much effort? Well forget it! With this easy plan you can get meals from the kitchen to the table in just half an hour a day!

It's so simple to follow: each day choose one breakfast, one light meal and one main meal. Vary your choices to ensure you get a range of nutrients. In total, your three meals will take no longer than 30 minutes to prepare and cook. As well as your meals, eat unlimited amounts of veg (see the *Free Vegetables* box).

■ Have 275ml/¹/₂pt skimmed milk a day on its own or in drinks, or 2 small pots of diet yoghurt instead. On top of what's in these recipes, this will provide essential calcium.
■ Have unlimited amounts of water, tea and coffee (with milk from the allowance), diet fizzy drinks and squash and herb teas.
■ Three meals plus the milk allowance and one 250-calorie snack gives 1,250 calories a day, suitable if you have less than 1st to lose. Between 1st and 3st to lose? Have an extra 250 calories a day from the veg list opposite. More than 3st to lose? Have an extra 500 calories a day by choosing three snacks.

HOW MUCH WEIGHT WILL I LOSE?

Around 1lb to 2lb a week, maybe more in the first weeks due to losing water as well as fat. In 2 weeks you can expect to lose up to 7lb.

BREAKFASTS
200 CALORIES

Ready in 5 minutes or less!

Summer fruits & yoghurt
Mix 75g/3oz each of the following: strawberries, blueberries, blackberries and blackcurrants. Serve with 1 small pot low-fat plain yogurt.

Bran and apricot cereal
Serve 25g/1oz bran cereal with 150ml/¹/₄pt skimmed milk and 3 chopped dried apricots.

Croissant & hot choc
Warm a 40g/1¹/₂oz croissant. Serve with 2 level tsp unsweetened jam. Plus 1 sachet low-fat hot chocolate.

Fruit salad
Serve 250g/9oz canned fruit cocktail in fruit juice with 1 small pot low-fat plain yoghurt.

Peanut butter roll
Top 1 toasted soft white bread roll with 2 level tsp peanut butter.

LIGHT MEALS
300 CALORIES

Ready in 10 minutes or less!

Filled pitta
Fill 1 warm wholemeal pitta with 'free' salad and:
■ 150g/5oz cottage cheese or
■ 40g/1¹/₂oz houmous or

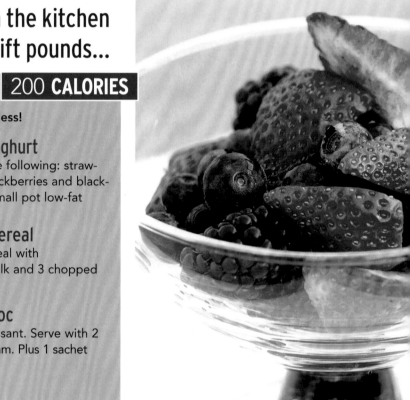

Dip into delicious summer fruits

■ 25g/1oz taramasalata or
■ 75g/3oz tuna canned in brine or water, drained and mixed with 1 level tbsp reduced-calorie mayonnaise.

Cheese Ploughman's
Serve 40g/1¹/₂oz crusty white bread with 40g/1¹/₂oz reduced-fat Cheddar cheese, 'free' salad, 1 apple and 1 level tbsp sweet pickle.

a day diet

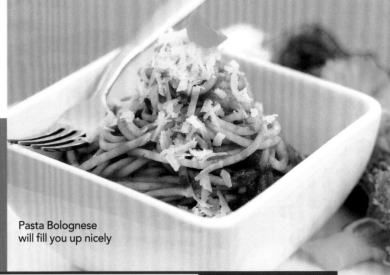

Pasta Bolognese
will fill you up nicely

MAIN MEALS

400 CALORIES

Ready in 15 minutes or less!

Steak sandwich
Grill a 100g/3½oz lean thin-sliced steak for 3 minutes on each side (or to taste). Serve in 75g/3oz ciabatta bread, sliced in half, with 1 level tbsp horseradish and 'free' salad.

Pasta Bolognese
Boil 65g/2½oz fresh pasta for 4 minutes and heat ½ x 375g pack fresh Bolognese sauce. Serve with 1 level tbsp grated Parmesan cheese and 'free' veg.

Grilled cod and new potatoes & peach
Boil 275g/10oz halved baby new potatoes for 10 minutes. Top a 150g/5oz cod fillet with 1 level tsp low-fat spread and lemon juice. Grill under medium heat for 10 minutes. Serve with potatoes and 'free' veg. Plus 1 peach.

Ratatouille and couscous
Place 50g/2oz couscous in a bowl and just cover with boiling water. Allow to stand for 2 minutes, season with black pepper. Heat a 390g can Ratatouille Provençale. Serve with 'free' salad.

Tuna and bean salad
Mix 75g/3oz tuna canned in brine with 75g/3oz canned mixed beans, ½ sliced medium avocado and 'free' salad. Toss with 2tbsp fat-free vinaigrette, serve with 25g/1oz crusty bread.

Wafer thin ham baguette
Slice 75g/3oz baguette in half and top with 1 level tsp low-fat spread. Fill with 40g/1½oz wafer-thin smoked ham and 'free' salad.

Spaghetti pesto
Boil 50g/2oz fresh egg spaghetti for 3 minutes, drain, mix with 1 level tbsp pesto sauce. Top with 1 level tbsp grated Parmesan cheese and serve with 'free' salad.

SNACKS

250 CALORIES

- 25g/1oz breakfast cereal with 150ml/¼pt skimmed milk. Plus 150ml/¼pt unsweetened orange juice and a small pot diet yoghurt.
- 1 toasted teacake with 1 level tsp each low-fat spread and unsweetened jam.
- 2 toasted crumpets with 1 level tbsp peanut butter.
- 1 bagel with 25g/1oz low-fat soft cheese.
- 150g/5oz ready-prepared rice salad.
- 200g/7oz ready-prepared pasta salad.
- 50g/2oz chocolate.
- 2 chocolate mini rolls.
- 50g/2oz bag nuts and raisins.
- 125ml/4½floz glass red or dry white wine, 275ml/½pt lager, beer or cider or 2 x 25ml measured spirit with a diet mixer plus 1 small packet crisps.

FREE VEGETABLES: EAT AS MUCH AS YOU LIKE!

As well as your meal choices, you may eat unlimited amounts of fruit, and the following vegetables. Don't add fat such as oil, butter, margarine, low-fat spread or oily dressings, though: Artichokes, asparagus, aubergines, beansprouts, broccoli, Brussels sprouts, cabbage, carrots, cauliflower, celery, chicory, courgettes, cucumber, fennel, garlic, gherkins, green beans, leeks, lettuce, mangetout, marrow, mushrooms, onions, peppers, pumpkins, radish, spinach, spring greens, swede, tomatoes, turnip and watercress.

Drop two dress sizes for summer

Make the most of the warmer summer weather, when many seasonal fruits and vegetables, such as strawberries, asparagus and new potatoes are available. Although you can buy most types of fruit and vegetables all year-round, buying in season means you get more for your money and they're often more flavoursome. So we've designed meal plans and recipes that make the most of the fruit and veg about during spring and summer, to bring you a diet packed full of a variety of nutrients. It should keep you feeling energised and healthy. We've also made the following recipes as easy as possible to prepare – leaving you more time to enjoy the warmer weather.

FEATURE: BRIGID MCKEVITH. PHOTOGRAPHY: REBECCA LACEY. STYLING: MAIRA ZOKAS. HAIR AND MAKE-UP: BRITTA D

Here's what to do

- Each day have one breakfast, one light meal and one main meal, plus your milk allowance (see below). Vary your meal choices to get a range of nutrients.
- Every day you should have 275ml/½pt skimmed milk for tea and coffee, or to drink on its own (as well as any milk that appears in the meals). You may have 2 small pots of diet yoghurt instead. Milk and yoghurt are sources of essential calcium so don't miss this out.
- The basic diet and milk allowance provide 1,000 calories per day. If you have less than 1st to lose, you should be on 1,250 calories a day, so have another 250 calories split between a morning and an afternoon snack. If you have between 1st and 3st to lose, you need another 500 calories a day, and if you have 3st or more to lose you should eat an extra 800 calories a day. Men should add an extra 250 calories to these figures. Make up these calories with snacks (either from those listed or calorie count your own) or by increasing your portion sizes.
- In addition to three meals and snacks, you may also have unlimited amounts of most vegetables (see 'Free vegetables'). But, remember, don't add any kind of fat during or after cooking.
- You may drink unlimited amounts of water (try for at least 2ltr a day), black tea and coffee, herbal teas, Bovril, Marmite and 'diet' or low-calorie soft drinks.
- Keep active. Exercise will help you lose weight and tone up. Our calorie allowances presume you're exercising for 30 minutes three times a week, so if you're not doing this, cut down by 250 calories a day.
NOTE: all teaspoon (tsp) and tablespoon (tbsp) measurements should be level.

How much weight will I lose?

Follow this diet for six weeks and you can expect to lose 1st – enough to drop a dress size. In the long term, aim for a weekly loss of 1lb to 2lb each week, although it's common to lose more than this when you first start your diet due to a loss of water as well as fat.

Free vegetables

You may eat unlimited amounts of the following vegetables: artichokes, asparagus, aubergines, bean sprouts, broccoli, Brussels sprouts, cabbage, carrots, cauliflower, celery, chicory, courgettes, cucumber, fennel, garlic, gherkins, green beans, leeks, lettuce, mangetout, marrow, mushrooms, onions, peppers, pumpkins, radish, spinach, spring greens, swede, tomatoes, turnip and watercress.

BREAKFASTS All serve 1
(250 calories)

Breakfast is a vital start to any day, no matter what the season. It's also a great opportunity to get at least one serving of the five portions of fruit and veg we should have every day.

1. BERRY MUESLI
Grate ½ small apple and mix with25g/1oz rolled oats and 1 walnut, finely chopped. Add 275ml/½pt skimmed milk and a small handful (about 5) raspberries.

2. BREAKFAST SMOOTHIE
Blend together 150ml/¼pt skimmed milk, 1tbsp low-fat plain yoghurt, 1 small banana and 2tbsp unsweetened museli.

3. MARMITE MUFFIN
Lightly toast 1 English muffin. Spread thinly with Marmite then top with 1 tomato, sliced, and freshly ground black pepper. Plus 1 medium apple.

4. PANCAKE AND HONEY
Warm 1 Scotch pancake, top with 1tbsp low-fat plain yoghurt and 1tsp honey. Plus 150ml/¼pt glass unsweetened orange juice.

5. BACON SANDWICH
Trim and grill 2 rashers lean back bacon. Serve between 2 slices wholemeal bread, thinly spread with tomato ketchup. Plus 1 satsuma.

If you want to get slim for your holiday, pack your diet with fresh fruit and vegetables, and every six weeks you could drop a dress size

LIGHT MEALS All serve 1

(300 calories)

Light summer meals don't have to mean just lettuce! Salads can be colourful and nutritious – and for a balanced and more filling meal you need to include ingredients such as wholemeal bread, pasta, rice or pulses. Fruits, nuts and seeds can also add variety, texture and flavour.

1. CHICKPEA AND TUNA SALAD

Mix $\frac{1}{2}$ x 410g can chickpeas with 50g/2oz tuna canned in brine, drained and flaked. Add $\frac{1}{2}$ small red onion and $\frac{1}{2}$ small cucumber, both finely diced, and 4 cherry tomatoes, halved. Dress with 1tsp chopped coriander, the juice of $\frac{1}{2}$ lemon, salt and pepper.

2. TUSCAN BREAD SALAD

Thinly slice 1in cucumber, sprinkle with salt and leave to stand in a colander for 15 minutes. Meanwhile lightly toast 2 thick slices wholemeal bread from a large loaf. Allow to cool then rip into bite-sized pieces. Mix the cucumber with 1 large tomato, thinly sliced, and the bread. Dress with 1tsp olive oil and the juice of $\frac{1}{2}$ lemon. Stand for 15 minutes before eating. Plus 125g pot diet yoghurt.

3. SPAGHETTI SALAD

Cook 65g/$2\frac{1}{2}$oz spaghetti according to packet instructions then rinse in cold water. Tip into a bowl, add a few sprays of one-calorie oil and mix in to avoid sticking. Add 1 carrot, peeled and grated, 1 celery stick, sliced, and 1 handful bean sprouts. Mix 1tsp smooth peanut butter with 1tsp hot water, 1tsp soya sauce and $\frac{1}{3}$tsp chilli flakes. Coat the pasta and vegetables.

4. ITALIAN PICNIC ROLL

Cut the lid off 1 small crusty roll and remove some bread from the centre. Rub the inside with a cut garlic clove. Spread 1tsp tapenade (olive paste) over the inside of the roll then layer 50g/2oz ricotta cheese, basil leaves, lettuce and sliced tomato, finishing with a layer of ricotta cheese. Replace the lid, wrap and weigh down. Leave for a few hours in the fridge to allow the flavours to seep into the bread.

5. GAZPACHO SOUP

Purée 410g can of tomatoes. Add 1 clove garlic, crushed; 1 small onion, diced; 1in cucumber, peeled and diced; $\frac{1}{2}$ medium red pepper, chopped; a dash of olive oil; and a dash of vinegar. Season with pepper and serve chilled with 1 small crusty brown roll. Plus 1 large banana.

6. MEXICAN WRAP

Spread 1 wheat tortilla with 3tbsp red kidney beans, mashed. Add free salad, then top with 1tbsp low-fat sour cream and 1tbsp guacamole. Roll up and serve with more salad.

7. MINI PIZZA

Top 75g/3oz medium-sized wholemeal pitta, uncut, with 1tbsp cranberry sauce. Add $\frac{1}{2}$ small onion, diced, and 20g/$\frac{3}{4}$oz brie, cut into chunks. Grill until cheese is melted and bubbling. Serve with free salad.

8. RICE SALAD

Cook 40g/$1\frac{1}{2}$oz long grain rice in boiling water. Drain and cool. Add 1tbsp sultanas, 1 slice pineapple, $\frac{1}{2}$ red pepper, 5 cashew nuts and 1tbsp reduced-calorie salad dressing. Plus 1 medium orange.

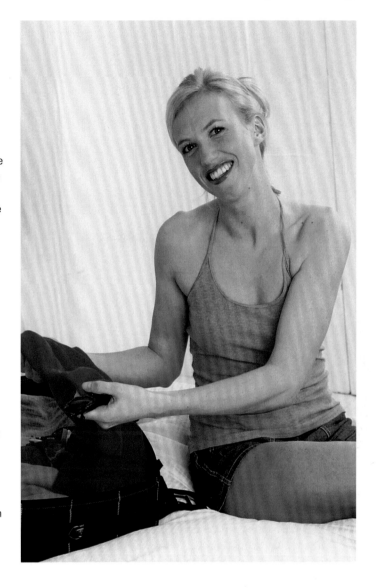

9. SALMON AND DILL PASTA

Cook 65g/$2\frac{1}{2}$oz pasta shapes. Mix with 50g/2oz smoked salmon, 2tbsp low-fat fromage frais and 1tsp fresh dill. Serve hot with free vegetables.

10. CHICKEN SALAD

Dice 100g/$3\frac{1}{2}$oz grilled chicken into bite-sized chunks. Add to cos lettuce, mangetout and cherry tomatoes. Top with croutons of 1 slice wholemeal toast. Dress salad with 1tsp pesto mixed with 1tbsp low-fat plain yoghurt.

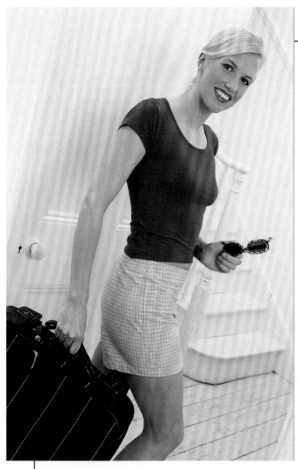

MAIN MEALS All serve 4
(350 calories per serving)

Many of these recipes, such as the stir-fried Thai prawn curry, are designed for speed. Others, such as the kebabs, can be cooked on the barbecue. Add more free veg to any of the dishes if you're feeling peckish.

1. LAMB KEBABS
Marinate 400g/14oz lean lamb, diced, with 1 garlic clove, crushed, 1tbsp tomato purée (diluted with 1tbsp water) and chopped rosemary. Cut 2 small onions into chunks. Thread the lamb and onion onto skewers and grill, brushing with remaining marinade. Serve with 4 x 40g/1$^{1}/_{2}$oz wholemeal pitta breads and 1tsp low-fat plain yoghurt.

2. THAI PRAWN CURRY
Cook 25g/1oz white rice per person. Purée 4tsp coriander leaves, 1tsp grated ginger, the juice of 1 lemon and 2 garlic cloves, crushed, adding water to make a paste. Dry-fry the paste in a wok for a few minutes then add 250g/9oz green beans, 250g/9oz baby corn and 400g/14oz prawns. Cook for two minutes then add 250ml/9floz coconut milk. Serve with the rice. Plus tropical fruit salad (see 'Exotic fruit').

3. PORK WITH MANGO SALSA
Boil 175g/6oz new potatoes per person. Mix 1 ripe mango, finely diced, 2 spring onions, chopped, and the juice of $^{1}/_{2}$ lime. Grill 450g/1lb pork fillet under a medium heat for 20 minutes. Serve with the salsa and potatoes, topped with 4tsp low-fat spread.

4. COUSCOUS WITH ROAST VEGETABLES
Put 4 courgettes, 1 aubergine and 4 carrots, all cut into chunks, into a tin sprayed with one-calorie spray oil. Roast at 220°C/425°F/ gas mark 7 for 25 minutes. In a saucepan, bring 115ml/4floz water to the boil. Tip in 115g/4oz couscous, stir, cover and stand for 15 minutes. Mix in 1 garlic clove, crushed, 1tbsp chopped parsley, 2tsp lemon juice and 4tsp pine nuts. Mix well. Serve with the veg and free salad. Plus 1 small banana.

5. TOFU AND APRICOT KEBABS
In a bowl, mix 1tbsp olive oil with 1tsp dried oregano. Add 200g/7oz tofu, diced, 4 dried apricots, halved, 4 prunes, halved, and the juice and zest of 1 lemon. Season and mix. Thread the tofu, apricots and prunes onto skewers. Grill, brushing with the marinade, until golden. Serve with 50g/2oz bulgar wheat cooked according to packet instructions mixed with 410g can chickpeas.

6. CHICKEN SESAME DRUMSTICKS
Skin 8 drumsticks and moisten with water. Mix 1tsp sesame seeds with 2tbsp plain flour in a plastic bag. Shake 2 drumsticks at a time in the bag to coat. Place on a roasting dish sprayed with one-calorie spray oil. Cook at 200°C/400°F/gas mark 6 for 20 minutes. Boil 675g/1$^{1}/_{2}$lb new potatoes and add 2tbsp fat-free dressing. Serve with the chicken and free vegetables.

7. BEEF FAJITAS WITH RICE
Cut 800g/1$^{3}/_{4}$lb fillet steak into strips and cook under a hot grill, along with 1 small onion and 1 green pepper, both cut into chunks. Divide into 4 warmed wheat tortillas and top each with 1tsp reduced-fat sour cream. Serve with free vegetables and 400g/14oz brown rice, cooked.

8. BAKED FISHCAKES
Poach 250g/9oz cod, then cool and flake. Mix with 400g/14oz potatoes, boiled and mashed with 1tbsp skimmed milk and 1tbsp chopped parsley. Shape into eight cakes and put in the fridge for 20 minutes. Spray with one-calorie spray oil and bake at 190°C/ 375°F/gas mark 5 for 15 minutes. Serve with 4 x 115g/4oz baked potatoes, topped with 1tsp low-fat spread and 1tbsp peas.

9. BAKED CHICKEN AND APRICOTS
Place 4 x 65g/2$^{1}/_{2}$oz skinless chicken breasts in the middle of four foil squares. Top each with $^{1}/_{2}$ fresh apricot and 2tsp goat's cheese, and wrap up in the foil. Bake at 190°C/375°F/ gas mark 5 for 20 minutes and serve with 2 x 410g cans cooked chickpeas, mashed with 1tbsp olive oil and the cooking liquid.

10. BLACK BEAN CURRY
Lightly sauté 1 onion and $^{1}/_{2}$ butter nut squash, diced. Add 1 garlic clove, crushed, and 1tbsp curry powder and fry for one minute. Add 410g can cooked black-eye beans and 250ml/9floz vegetable stock. Simmer for 20 minutes and serve with 4 x 75g/3oz wholemeal pitta breads.

SNACKS

50-CALORIE SNACKS
- 1 medium orange
- 1 medium apple
- Small handful of popcorn
- 1 jaffa cake biscuit
- Selection of exotic fruit

150-CALORIE SNACKS
- 25g/1oz bag of Bombay mix
- 2 x 8g meringues with 60g pot fat-free fromage frais and a large handful of strawberries
- Milky Way or 2-finger Kit-Kat
- 2 water crackers and a small matchbox-size chunk of blue cheese

- Fruit kebabs: thread 5 marshmallows cut in half, 1 kiwi fruit, chopped into chunks, and $1/2$ small banana, sliced, onto toothpicks

250-CALORIE SNACKS
- Small 35g bag of tortilla chips with salsa made from 1 small onion, finely diced, 1 small tomato, roughly diced, 1tsp fresh coriander and a squeeze of lemon juice
- 50g/2oz bag dry roasted peanuts
- 1 small wholemeal crusty roll with 1tsp heaped chocolate nut spread
- 65g/$2^1/2$oz waffle warmed and served with 1tsp honey

EXOTIC FRUIT

As with all fruit, exotic fruit are low in fat, making them great snacks and bases for summery desserts. Many can also be incorporated into savoury dishes. While you can get exotic fruit all year round in most supermarkets, they're in more bountiful supply over the summer months, so make the most of them.

GUAVA
The guava is quite small and round or pear-shaped with a thin, greenish-yellow skin and white, yellow-pink or red flesh. You can eat the whole fruit, including the seeds at the centre.
7 calories per 25g/1oz

PASSION FRUIT
The leathery, purple-brown skin becomes brittle and wrinkled when ripe. Inside, the jelly-like pulp has a lemony, tart flavour and contains edible small, black seeds. Cut in half and scoop out the pulp with a spoon.
5 calories per fruit

MANGO
Delicious in fruit salads or on their own, there are many different types of mango. Peel and de-stone before eating.
85 calories per medium fruit

PAPAYA (PAWPAW)
This fruit resembles a pear with yellow or orange skin when ripe. It has a sweet flavour with small, inedible black seeds in the centre like a melon. Peel and remove seeds before eating.
10 calories per 25g/1oz flesh

EXOTIC FRUIT SNACKS

TROPICAL FRUIT SALAD (65 calories)
Chop 1 large slice fresh pineapple and 1 kiwi fruit into chunks and serve with $1/2$ passion fruit.

TROPICAL SMOOTHIE (145 calories)
Blend 150ml/$1/4$pt skimmed milk with 1tbsp low-fat plain yoghurt, $1/2$ small banana, sliced, and 40g/$1^1/2$oz papaya, diced. Add 1tsp honey and serve in a chilled glass.

HOW TO **UP YOUR PORTION SIZE**

If you prefer to increase the portion size of some of your meals rather than eating snacks, use the following table to help 'spend' your calories:

MENU ITEM	ADD 150 CALORIES	ADD 250 CALORIES
Chickpea and tuna salad	+ 2tbsp chickpeas into the salad	+ 3tbsp chickpeas into the salad
Tuscan bread salad	+ 1 thick slice bread + 1tsp olive oil	+ 2 thick slices bread + 1tsp olive oil
Spaghetti salad	+ 50g/2oz spaghetti, raw weight	+ 75g/3oz spaghetti, raw weight
Italian picnic roll	+ 1 large crusty roll +25g ricotta cheese	+ 1 small roll + 50g/2oz ricotta + $1/2$tsp tapenade
Mexican wrap	+ $1/2$ tortilla wrap + 1tbsp red kidney beans, mashed	+ 1 tortilla wrap + 3tbsp red kidney beans, mashed
Mini pizza	Use large (100g/$3^1/2$oz) pitta bread instead + 20g/$3/4$oz cheese	+ medium (75g/3oz) pitta + 20g/$3/4$oz cheese
Rice salad	Double the amount of rice used	Double the recipe
Salmon pasta	Use 100g/$3^1/2$oz raw pasta and 75g/3oz salmon instead	Use 115g/4oz raw pasta and 75g/3oz salmon instead
Chicken salad	+ 1 thick slice wholemeal toast for croutons	+ 2 thick slices of toast for croutons + $1^1/2$ medium (100g/$3^1/2$oz) chicken breasts
Lamb kebabs	Use 75g/3oz medium pitta bread instead	+ 2 x small (40g/$1^1/2$oz) pitta breads
Thai prawn curry	Double the amount of rice used	Triple the amount of rice used
Pork with mango salsa	Double the amount of potatoes used	Triple the amount of potatoes used
Couscous with roasted veg	Double the amount of couscous used	Triple the amount of couscous used
Tofu and apricot kebabs	Double the amount of bulgar wheat used	Double the amount of wheat and chickpeas used
Chicken sesame drumsticks	Double the amount of potatoes used	Triple the amount of potatoes used
Beef fajitas	Double the amount of rice used	Triple the amount of rice used
Baked fishcakes	Use medium (175g/6oz) potatoes per person	Use 2 medium (175g/6oz) potatoes per person
Baked chicken and apricots	+ 3tbsp chickpeas	Double the amount of chickpeas used
Black bean curry	+ $1/2$ x medium (75g/3oz) pitta bread	+ medium (75g/3oz) pitta bread

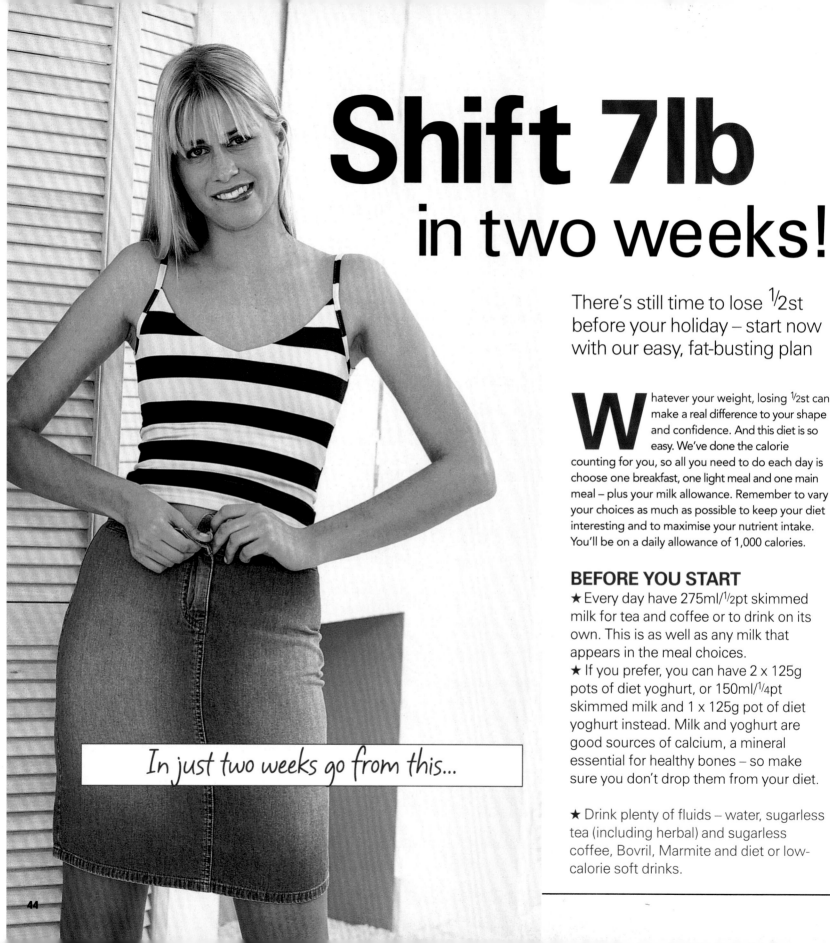

Shift 7lb
in two weeks!

There's still time to lose $\frac{1}{2}$st before your holiday – start now with our easy, fat-busting plan

Whatever your weight, losing $\frac{1}{2}$st can make a real difference to your shape and confidence. And this diet is so easy. We've done the calorie counting for you, so all you need to do each day is choose one breakfast, one light meal and one main meal – plus your milk allowance. Remember to vary your choices as much as possible to keep your diet interesting and to maximise your nutrient intake. You'll be on a daily allowance of 1,000 calories.

BEFORE YOU START
★ Every day have 275ml/$\frac{1}{2}$pt skimmed milk for tea and coffee or to drink on its own. This is as well as any milk that appears in the meal choices.
★ If you prefer, you can have 2 x 125g pots of diet yoghurt, or 150ml/$\frac{1}{4}$pt skimmed milk and 1 x 125g pot of diet yoghurt instead. Milk and yoghurt are good sources of calcium, a mineral essential for healthy bones – so make sure you don't drop them from your diet.

★ Drink plenty of fluids – water, sugarless tea (including herbal) and sugarless coffee, Bovril, Marmite and diet or low-calorie soft drinks.

In just two weeks go from this...

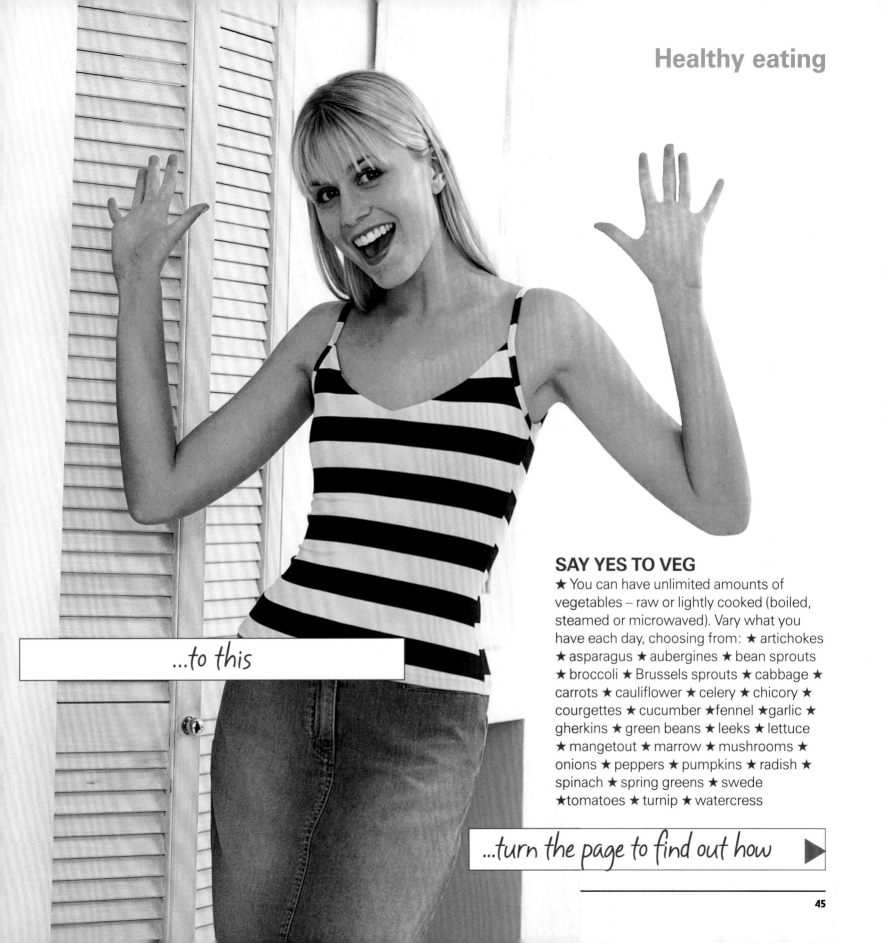

...to this

SAY YES TO VEG
★ You can have unlimited amounts of vegetables – raw or lightly cooked (boiled, steamed or microwaved). Vary what you have each day, choosing from: ★ artichokes ★ asparagus ★ aubergines ★ bean sprouts ★ broccoli ★ Brussels sprouts ★ cabbage ★ carrots ★ cauliflower ★ celery ★ chicory ★ courgettes ★ cucumber ★fennel ★garlic ★ gherkins ★ green beans ★ leeks ★ lettuce ★ mangetout ★ marrow ★ mushrooms ★ onions ★ peppers ★ pumpkins ★ radish ★ spinach ★ spring greens ★ swede ★tomatoes ★ turnip ★ watercress

...turn the page to find out how ▶

Breakfasts
(250 calories)

The cereal breakfast
150ml/¼pt unsweetened orange or grapefruit juice, 40g/1½oz non sugar-coated cereal such as branflakes, cornflakes or muesli with 150ml/¼pt skimmed milk.

The fruit and yoghurt breakfast
150g pot 0% fat Greek yoghurt topped with 1 medium banana, sliced, and 1tbsp runny honey.

The smoothie breakfast
Put 115ml/4floz skimmed milk, 3tbsp low-fat natural yoghurt, 1 small banana, 1 small, skinned peach and 10 hulled strawberries into a blender and blend until frothy. Pour into a glass and drink immediately.

The cooked breakfast
2 medium eggs, beaten, with 1tbsp water and seasoning. Heat 1tsp oil in a non-stick frying pan, pour in the egg mixture and cook for about one minute with 50g/2oz sliced mushrooms, until the base is set. Plus 1 medium slice wholemeal toast.

On the move breakfast
200ml bottle freshly squeezed orange juice, plus 1 Kellogg's Special K Bar, and 15 grapes.

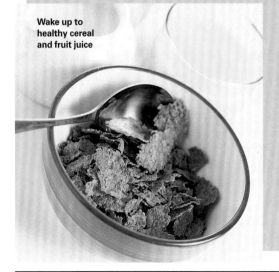

Wake up to healthy cereal and fruit juice

Light meals
(300 calories)
Salad-based meals
★ Mix raw veg with 2tbsp low-fat French dressing. Add a small can tuna in brine, drained, flaked and sprinkled with lemon juice, and 1tbsp capers. Serve with 3 Original or Dark Rye Ryvita and 1 medium apple.
VARIATION:
Instead of tuna and capers, try 1 medium hard-boiled egg, chopped and mixed with 1tbsp reduced-calorie salad cream; or 50g/2oz reduced-fat Cheshire cheese, crumbled.

Sandwich-based meals
★ Spread 1 granary roll with low-fat spread, fill with 50g/2oz wafer-thin turkey. Top with 2tbsp cranberry sauce. Serve with cherry tomatoes. Finish with 125g pot diet yoghurt, and 1 kiwi.
VARIATION:
Instead of turkey, try 4 reduced fat cheese triangles.

★ 2 medium slices wholemeal bread, covered with low-fat spread, 40g/1½oz reduced-fat Edam cheese, sliced, and 1 medium apple, sliced. Serve with salad of raw vegetables.

★ Fill 1 small pitta bread with 50g/2oz low-fat liver pâté. Serve with salad and 20 grapes.
VARIATION:
Instead of liver pâté, try 50g/2oz spinach and soft cheese pâté.

Readymade sandwiches
★ Boots Feta Cheese Flatbread.
★M&S Chicken No Mayonnaise Sandwich.
★ Tesco Healthy Eating Bacon, Lettuce and Tomato.

Eating out
Pizza Hut – 2 slices The Edge pizza and salad bowl.
Pub lunch – vegetable lasagne with salad.
McDonald's – 1 cheeseburger and 1 Diet Coke.

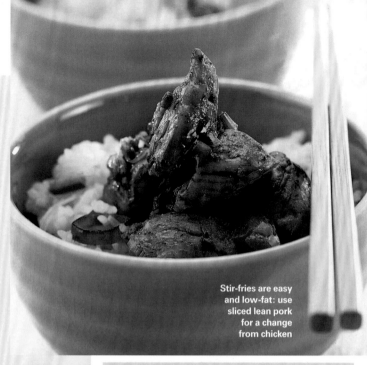

Stir-fries are easy and low-fat: use sliced lean pork for a change from chicken

Main meals
(350 calories)
Sausages and mash
Grill 3 low-fat, small sausages (90g/3¼oz for 3 meat sausages, 150g/5oz for 3 vegetarian). Boil 150g/5oz potatoes for about 20 minutes, mash them with a little mustard to taste, and serve with veg. Follow with a bowl of 100g/3½oz fresh fruit salad.

Easy stir-fry
Thinly slice 100g/3½oz skinless chicken breast, stir-fry for a few minutes before adding vegetables that are suitable for stir-frying. Season with 1tbsp soy sauce. Serve with 50g/2oz boiled white rice (uncooked weight), followed by 100g/3½oz strawberries topped with 1tbsp low-fat natural yoghurt.
VARIATION:
Instead of chicken, use 100g/ 3½oz lean pork or 100g/3½oz shelled prawns or 100g/3½oz tofu, cubed.

Baked potato supper
Serve 100g/3½oz roasted chicken, with 1 medium jacket potato, and vegetables. Plus a large piece of watermelon.
VARIATION:
Instead of chicken, you can use 2 grilled Quorn fillets.

Savoury mince

Dry-fry 100g/3½oz extra-lean minced beef or minced Quorn, with a small onion, chopped, for two to three minutes until the meat is brown and onion soft. Stir in 200g/7oz canned tomatoes and a pinch of mixed herbs. Simmer for 25 minutes until the sauce has thickened. Season. Top with 150g/5oz mashed potatoes. Plus 1 peach.
VARIATION:
Instead of mash, you can serve this dish with 50g/2oz boiled pasta (uncooked weight), and vegetables or a side salad.

Quick kebabs

Cube 100g/3½oz skinless chicken breast and thread on to skewers alternating with onions, peppers and tomatoes. Grill for 10 minutes or until cooked, turning regularly. Serve with 50g/2oz boiled rice (uncooked weight), and a side salad. Finish with 1 slice melon, cubed, and mixed with 2tbsp low-fat natural yoghurt.
VARIATION:
Instead of chicken, use 150g/5oz thick cod fillet or 100g/3½oz tofu, cubed.

Summer salad

Serve 100g/3½oz lean ham with a salad or vegetables. Drizzle with 2tbsp low-fat French dressing. Eat with 1 crusty roll, followed by 100g/ 3½oz raspberries topped with 1tbsp low-fat, natural yoghurt.
VARIATION:
Instead of ham, try 100g/3½oz cold chicken, or Quorn (both roasted).

Ready meals

★ 360g/12oz M&S Count on Us Lasagne.
★ 340g/12oz Tesco Healthy Eating Tuna and Pasta Bake.
★ 300g/11oz Quorn lasagne, followed by 25g/1oz low-fat soft cheese, and 2 crispbreads.

Serve all of the above ready meals with a side salad, plus 1 medium nectarine.

POST-EXERCISE REFUELLERS

If you already exercise regularly you'll need to do some fast refuelling as soon as possible after you finish. What this does is to replace the fuel in your muscles that you've just used up, so that you have enough energy for the next session. Choose from the selected tasty treats below – and there's no need to include them in your calorie allowance! Don't forget to keep your fluid intake up as well. It's important to make sure that you always drink plenty of water before, during and after exercise.

★ 3 jaffa cakes
★ 1 Jordans Frusli Bar
★ 1 McVities Go Ahead Apple Bake
★ 1 currant bun
★ 1 large banana
★ 6 dried apricots

DAMAGE LIMITATION

No matter how good your intentions, sometimes you get a craving for something that just won't go away. Nip it in the bud by having a 'taster', as well as your daily 1,000-calorie allowance – the secret is to enjoy it and move on. If you resist a craving it can become a full-blown binge, and that will wreck all the good work you've done so far. Feel the urge? Try whichever one suits the occasion. Don't have more than one a day, though, or you won't shift those pounds!
You can take your pick from 1 pub measure of spirits and low-calorie mixer, or one small glass dry white wine, or 70g carton M&S Count on Us Chocolate Mousse, or 1 Mini Babybel Light with 2 breadsticks or 2 After Eight Mints.

GET PHYSICAL, BURN CALORIES

Increase your physical activity level and not only will you burn more calories, you'll also start to tone up your body, and that in itself will make you feel and look better.

Number of calories burned by half an hour of exercising*

Walking briskly	180
Cycling (pedalling fast)	195
Dancing (energetically)	195
Tennis	210
Swimming (gently)	255
Lifting weights	165
Cycling in the gym (moderate effort)	120
Squash	420

*Figures based on 10st 3lb female.

FEATURE: JANE GRIFFIN. PHOTOGRAPHY: MARTIN SHAW

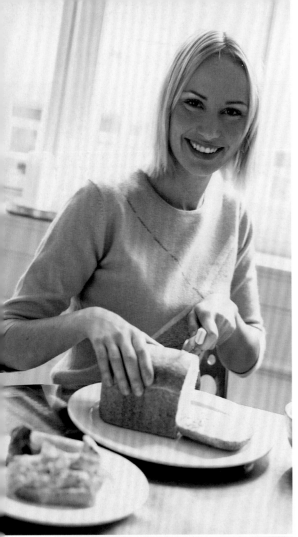

FEATURE: JENNETTE HIGGS

Your 'get back on track' diet

Breakfasts

300 calories

● **Fruity cereal**
40g/1½oz wholegrain cereal (for example, Weetabix, Branflakes, Wheatflakes, Shreddies, Shredded Wheat or malty flakes), topped with a medium banana, sliced, 10 fresh or frozen raspberries, strawberries or other fruit, and 175ml/6floz semi-skimmed milk.

● **Toast, low-fat yoghurt and fruit**
125g pot low-fat yoghurt, 1 thick slice wholemeal toast spread with 1tsp jam, honey or marmalade. Plus 125g/4½oz fruit salad made from fresh, frozen or canned fruit in natural juice (for example, sliced apple, satsuma, grapes and apricots canned in natural juice) or 2 small pieces fresh fruit.

We all have times when our diet goes off the rails – whether it's at a family party or a weekend away that turns into one giant binge! But don't worry – it needn't mean you've blown it – you just need a few days of firm guidance to get you back on track. Our four-day plan will help you shed newly-gained pounds, and restore your enthusiasm!

How do I follow this diet?

Each day choose one breakfast, one lunch and one dinner, plus one snack to give you a total of 1,250 calories. If you've really overindulged recently and now need to lose more than 1st you can add in an extra 150-calorie snack each day. **NB:** As the lunches and main meals are all 400 calories, you can interchange these to increase your choices. But the important thing is to stick with it, so read *7 Ways To Stop The Rot.*

Lunches

400 calories

● **Filled baguette and fresh strawberries**
Spread 75g/3oz French bread with 1tsp Dijon mustard and top with 50g/2oz lean ham plus 75g/3oz salad (for example, tomato, lettuce, cucumber, onion and carrot). Have 10 fresh strawberries topped with 1tbsp Greek style yoghurt and ½tsp sugar.

● **Quick couscous and bean salad**
Cook 50g/2oz couscous (dry weight), and drain. Mix with 1tsp coriander, freshly chopped, 40g/1½oz cucumber, finely chopped, 50g/2oz red pepper, finely chopped, and 100g/3½oz canned red kidney beans, drained. Cube 50g/2oz avocado, toss in 1tbsp lemon juice, drizzle with 1tsp olive oil, add to the cooled salad and mix. Mix 1tsp mint sauce jelly into 65g/2½oz very low-fat fromage frais and serve on the side with 5 cherry tomatoes.

● **Dips with oatcakes and crudités**
Make a quick dip by mixing 50g/2oz tuna, canned in oil, drained, with 30g/1¼oz reduced- fat houmous and ¼tsp chilli sauce or Tabasco. Serve with 2 x 30g/1¼oz oatcakes, 3 breadsticks, plus 1 apple, 1 carrot and 2 sticks of celery, cut into dipping sticks.

● **Tasty packed lunch standby – peanut butter or cream cheese sandwich and fruit or low-fat yoghurt**
Knock up a super-speedy sandwich with 2 medium slices wholemeal bread spread with 1tbsp peanut butter or 40g/1½oz low-fat cream cheese. Add 10 grapes to the sandwich, but leave them whole to prevent the bread turning soggy. Plus 1 small orange or apple and 125g pot low-fat yoghurt.

Dinners
400 calories

● **Peppery steak and vegetable mash**
Arrange 115g/4oz beef topside or pork steak with 125g/4^1/2oz peppers, quartered, in a shallow dish. Drizzle over 1tsp olive oil and sprinkle with 1tsp herbs. Grill on a medium heat and turn regularly until cooked. Peel and chop 125g/4^1/2oz potatoes, 1 carrot, 1 leek and 1 clove garlic. Boil until soft, then drain, leaving some liquid for moisture. Add 15g/^{1}/2oz low-fat soft cheese and mash. Serve with 125g/4^1/2oz French beans.

● **Pan-fried salmon**
Add 1tsp olive oil to a non-stick pan, heat and, when warm, add 1 clove garlic, chopped, plus 65g/2^1/2oz salmon steak. Sizzle for 2 minutes, then turn and add 200g/7oz spinach. Cover the pan and leave on a medium heat for 5 minutes. Toss the spinach in the fish juices, season and re-cover. Leave for 5 more minutes. Make a salad from 75g/3oz lettuce and 40g/1^1/2oz cucumber, and toss with a mix of 1tsp honey and 1tbsp lemon juice. Serve with 1 slice wholemeal bread. Plus 125g pot low-fat yoghurt.

● **Broccoli pasta bake**
Boil 40g/1^1/2oz (raw weight) cooked wholemeal pasta, and steam 125g/4^1/2oz broccoli until al dente. In an ovenproof dish, melt 50g/ 2oz low-fat soft cheese in a microwave with ^{1}/2 small onion, finely chopped, then mix in 100ml/ 4floz semi-skimmed milk, ^{1}/4tsp nutmeg, ^{1}/4tsp paprika pepper and black pepper. Mix the broccoli cooking water into the sauce. Add the broccoli and drained pasta, tossing all with the sauce. Sprinkle over ^{1}/3 of a Weetabix, crushed with 1tbsp fresh chopped basil, and cook in a medium oven for 10 minutes. Serve with 125g/ 4^1/2oz tomatoes tossed with a dressing of 1tsp olive oil, 1tbsp balsamic vinegar and 2tsp fresh mint.

● **Quick veggie stir-fry**
Heat 1tsp groundnut oil in a non-stick wok. Add 1 clove garlic, chopped, 1 small onion, chopped, and 25g/1oz peanuts, and cook for 1 min. Add 400g stir-fry veg, such as bean sprouts, mangetout and sliced peppers, plus 1tbsp orange juice to prevent sticking and 1tsp Chinese five spice powder. Toss and cook for 3 minutes. Add 1tbsp soy sauce, bring back to the boil and serve with 40g/1^1/2oz (raw weight) cooked basmati rice. Drink an extra 125ml/ 5floz semi-skimmed milk on the day you have this meal.

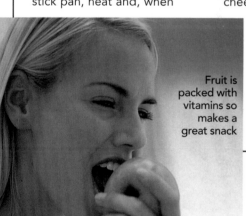

Fruit is packed with vitamins so makes a great snack

Snacks
150 calories

● **Apricot yoghurt**
Serve 125g/4^1/2oz apricots canned in natural juice with 125g pot low-fat fruit yoghurt.

● **Houmous and veg**
75g/3oz reduced-fat houmous with 2 sticks celery and 65g/2^1/2oz cucumber, quartered.

● **Wrap snack**
Spread a 40g/1^1/2oz tortilla wrap with 15g/^{1}/2oz

● **Banana and honey bagel**
Spread half a toasted bagel with ^{1}/2tsp honey and half a banana, sliced.

low-fat soft cheese plus ^{1}/3tsp Marmite. Top with 25g/1oz crispy lettuce and wrap up.

● **Wine**
225ml (a large glass) dry white wine.

● **Fruit 'n' nut**
20g/^{3}/4oz ready-to-eat apricots, cut into quarters with 20g/^{3}/4oz roasted peanuts or a handful of nuts and raisins.

● **Egg and tomato**
One medium boiled egg with 1 medium slice wholemeal toast for dipping; 1 medium tomato, quartered on the side.

7 ways to STOP THE ROT

Think about it: the fact that you're reading this is half the battle won – follow this plan to get back into the swing of things!

Make small cut backs – just a few hundred cals less a day is enough to stop you gaining any weight.

Plan your meals and snacks to help you avoid impulse eating.

Think about your overeating – why, what, when and how much, then use this plan to re-adjust your eating.

Normal portions are best – as large portion sizes is one of the major causes of obesity.

Exercise – even a brisk walk outside will help take your mind off food.

Watch the weight fall off – if your weight's shot up because of a few days of bingeing, follow this plan and you'll see it fall off almost as quickly. Don't let your body get used to this heavier new you – give it a healthy break and you'll soon recover your normal appetite.

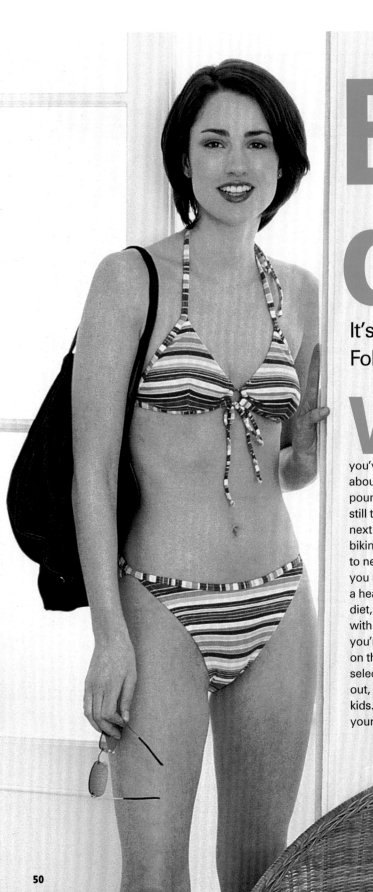

Bikini diet

Lose a stone in time for summer

It's never too late to get a body fit for the beach. Follow our easy diet and lose 1st in about six weeks.

We've all been there. The sun's reappeared and summer holidays are looming. But you've probably not done much about shedding those extra winter pounds yet. Don't despair, there's still time to lose a stone over the next six weeks, ready to fit into that bikini. And there's no need to resort to near-starvation regimes that do you no good in the long run. Here's a healthy and filling pick and mix diet, designed to suit busy lifestyles with great meal options whether you're at home or eating at work or on the move. We've even included a selection of options for the odd meal out, or trip to McDonald's with the kids. So, no more excuses, kick-start your healthy summer eating – today.

THE RULES

● Each day have one breakfast, one lunch, one evening meal and a 150-calorie snack (or more, depending on the weight you have to lose) plus your milk allowance.

● The basic diet, including allowances, allows you 1,250 calories per day, which is sufficient for those with up to 1st to lose. If you have between 1st and 3st to lose, you need an extra 250 calories a day. More than 3st to lose, add 550 calories a day. Men should add an extra 250 calories to these figures. Make up these calories from the snacks listed, or calorie count your own.

● Every day have 275ml/½pt skimmed milk, or two small pots of diet yoghurt, for calcium. Use this in tea and coffee, or to drink on its own (this is in addition to any milk that appears in the meals).

● You may eat unlimited amounts of 'free' vegetables and fruit. Just don't add any kind of fat during or after cooking. Don't overcook the vegetables and, where possible, cook them lightly in the microwave and

300 CALS
BREAKFAST AT HOME

● **WEEKEND BRUNCH** (SERVES 4)
Mash 240g/8^1/2oz cooked potatoes with 2tsp butter. Work 60g/2^1/2oz flour into the potatoes to make a stiff dough. Roll out and cut into 8 thick triangles. Heat 2tsp oil in a pan and cook the potato cakes over a low to medium heat until golden, then turn and cook the other side. Serve 2 potato cakes with 2 rashers lean back bacon, dry-fried, 4 small mushrooms, sliced and dry-fried, 1 tomato, grilled, 1tbsp baked beans and 100ml/3^1/2floz orange juice.

FEATURE: COLETTE KELLY. PHOTOGRAPHY: REBECCA LACEY. STYLING: MARIA ZOKAS. HAIR AND MAKE-UP: BRITTA D

● **CHEESE AND TOMATO CRUMPETS**
Toast 2 x 40g/1^1/2oz crumpets on both sides, spread each with 1tsp Marmite and 15g/^{1}/2oz low-fat soft cheese. Top with a sliced tomato, black pepper and just a pinch (^{1}/2tsp) Cheddar cheese, grated. Put under the grill until the cheese bubbles. Follow with ^{1}/2 grapefruit sprinkled with 1tsp sugar.

● **FRUIT SHAKE** (SERVES 2)
Blend 1 banana with 125ml/4^1/2floz low-fat natural bio yoghurt and 50g/2oz sugar-free muesli until the muesli is well ground. Add 425g/15oz unsweetened peaches canned in juice and blend until smooth. Store in the fridge and use within two days.

NB: Vary the flavour with different fruits and yoghurts, eg apricots with peach melba yoghurt; pears with cherry yoghurt; or blackberries with raspberry yoghurt.

● **BAGEL AND ORANGE JUICE**
Spread ^{1}/2 bagel (or wholemeal roll), toasted, with 25g/1oz low-fat soft cheese, and top with 1tsp honey and 1 small banana, sliced. Serve with 100ml/3^1/2floz unsweetened orange juice.

● **PANCAKE WITH FRESH FRUIT**
Spread 2 x 65g/2^1/2oz Scotch pancakes, toasted, with 1tsp jam or honey and top with summer fruits, eg blackcurrants, strawberries, blackberries and raspberries.

use any vegetable stock for gravy or sauces (it's full of vitamins). Quantities of salad and vegetables given in the recipes are given as a guide – you can eat larger quantities if they're in the 'free' vegetable list.
● You can drink unlimited water, black tea and coffee, herbal teas, Bovril, Marmite and low-calorie squashes and diet soft drinks. Aim for 2ltr of drinks a day.
● Spread your snacks and meals throughout the day and don't skip breakfast. Make sure you vary your meals to get the full range of nutrients you need for good health.
● On those days when you eat your main meal out, use the 650-calorie selections to guide your choices and for the rest of the day choose a breakfast option plus a lunch or a selection of snacks to make up your calorie total. So if you're on 1,250 calories, choose a breakfast plus two 150-calorie snacks, or one 250-calorie snack plus a 50-calorie snack, or a 300-calorie lunch.
● All meals serve one unless specified.
● Most important of all, aim to exercise for 30 minutes three to five times a week. Not only will it shift calories, but it'll help to tone your muscles at the same time. Think active and be active and you'll have less time to be thinking about food. If you're not doing the equivalent of 30 minutes three times a week, cut down by 250 calories a day.

300 CALS
BREAKFAST ON THE GO

● **TOAST, YOGHURT AND FRUIT**
1 thick slice wholemeal toast spread with 1tsp jam. Plus 1 fresh peach, sliced, topped with 125ml/4^1/2floz low-fat yoghurt.
● Or 125g pot low-fat yoghurt, 10 grapes, 1 Clementine and 1 small (50g/2oz) wholemeal roll, toasted, with 1tsp jam.

● **CEREAL AND FRUIT**
20g/3^1/2oz serving Bran Flakes plus 1 Weetabix, topped with 1 small banana, sliced, and 15g/^{1}/2oz raisins served with 150ml/^{1}/4pt skimmed milk.
● Or 200ml/7floz carton fruit juice, Kelloggs Nutri-Grain bar, plus 1 medium banana.
● **TOAST AND PEANUT BUTTER**
2 medium slices brown or wholemeal toast with ^{1}/2tbsp peanut butter on each and 1 orange.

300 CALS
LUNCH AT HOME

● **BAGUETTES** (SERVES 2)
Spread 40g/1^1/2oz low-fat soft cheese with chives or garlic into a part-baked baguette before cooking. Serve each half warm with 75g/3oz salad leaves and sliced tomatoes.
● Alternatively fill with 1tsp red pesto and 40g/1^1/2oz low-fat soft cheese, or 3tsp mustard and 25g/1oz finely chopped ham.
● **GREEK BEAN SALAD**
Toss 175g/6oz ready-prepared low-fat three-bean salad with 1 spring onion, chopped, and 25g/1oz feta cheese, cubed. Serve with 1 large tomato, sliced, and 1 thin slice wholemeal bread.

● **SAUSAGE AND MUSTARD SALAD**
Chop 1 sausage, grilled. Add to lettuce, watercress, cherry tomatoes and cucumber. Dress with 1tbsp wholegrain mustard, 1tbsp balsamic vinegar, and 1tsp honey. Serve with 50g/2oz granary bread.
● **BAKED BEANS ON TOAST**
Top 2 medium slices wholegrain toast with 75g/3oz baked beans, 115g/4oz low-fat cottage cheese and tomatoes.
● **NICOISE PASTA SALAD**
Mix 50g/2oz tuna canned in brine with 25g/1oz (dry weight) cooked pasta, 1 spring onion, chopped, ^{1}/2 red pepper, diced, and 3 black olives, sliced. Toss in 3tbsp 0% fat Greek yoghurt, 1tsp mustard, 1tsp honey, black pepper and lemon juice. Serve with 1 boiled egg, chopped, and chicory leaves.

300 CALS

READY-PREPARED SANDWICHES, SALADS AND WRAPS

Supermarkets, Marks & Spencer, Boots, delicatessens and BP garages all do a good range of healthy, low-calorie sandwiches, pasta bowls, wraps and salads. Look for those under 300 calories. As a general rule, keep down fat and calories by avoiding any that include mayonnaise and hard cheese.

BAKED POTATOES

Ask for a small potato without butter or mayonnaise. Stick to fillings such as ham and sweetcorn, baked beans, or tuna and peppers. Or ask for a plain potato with salad and reduced fat cheese triangles.

SOUPS

Stick to non-creamy soups, eg vegetable, tomato and basil, carrot and coriander, or wild mushroom. Finish with a piece of fresh fruit, eg 8 strawberries, 10 cherries, or 10 grapes.

SUSHI

Many supermarket chains sell sushi – a wonderfully filling mix of rice and fish. Look for packs under 300 calories.

SOME PACKED LUNCH IDEAS

- 4 Ryvitas and low-calorie soup, plus fruit.
- Tuna with bread roll or a piece of fruit.

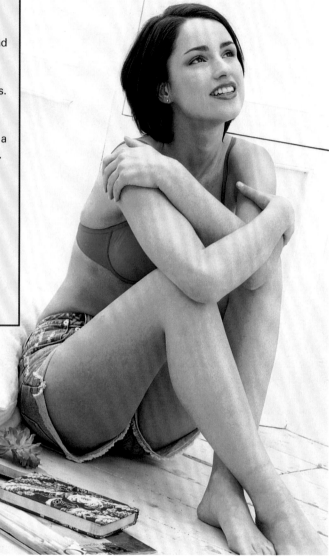

400 CALS

● HAM & SWEETCORN JACKETS

Bake a 175g/6oz potato. Scoop out the flesh and mix with 70g/3oz lean ham, chopped, 25g/1oz sweetcorn and 2tsp honey mustard. Refill the skin with the mix and return to the oven for five minutes. Serve with salad.

● PORK STEAK WITH RATATOUILLE AND NEW POTATOES (SERVES 2)

Heat 2tsp olive oil, add 1 small onion, sliced, 2 garlic cloves, crushed, and $^1/_2$ medium aubergine, 1 courgette and 1 pepper, all chopped. Cover and cook gently for one minute. Add 400g can chopped tomatoes, 1tsp dried mixed herbs and season. Simmer uncovered for 10 minutes. Serve over 2 x 75g/3oz (raw weight) pork steaks, trimmed and grilled, with 250g/9oz new potatoes.

● PASTA AND TUNA BAKE (SERVES 2)

Heat 1tsp oil and fry 1 onion and 2 garlic cloves, both finely chopped. Add 1 medium red pepper, chopped, 75g/3oz sweetcorn, 185g can tuna in brine, drained, 40g/1$^1/_2$oz very low-fat soft cheese, 2tsp dried tarragon and 150ml/$^1/_4$pt vegetable stock. Mix and cook in a pan for five minutes. Toss with 125g/4$^1/_2$oz (raw weight) cooked pasta and bake in a hot oven for five minutes. Serve with 175g/6oz broccoli.

● CHICKEN KORMA (SERVES 4)

Heat 1tsp oil and stir-fry 1 medium onion, chopped, 2 garlic cloves, crushed, and 450g/1lb lean chicken, diced, for five minutes. Mix in 2tbsp mild curry powder, 1tsp cumin, 1tbsp flour and 275ml/$^1/_2$pt chicken stock. Simmer gently until sauce thickens. Remove from the heat and stir in 275ml/$^1/_2$pt low-fat natural yoghurt, 25g/1oz sweet mango chutney and 2tbsp chopped coriander. Serve with 175g/6oz (dry weight) boiled rice, 225g/8oz courgettes, sliced, plus 275g/10oz mangetout, steamed.

GENERAL TIPS WHEN EATING OUT

- Always go for a salad-based starter instead of a dessert.
- Ask for dressings on the side, go easy on them and avoid mayo or blue cheese varieties.
- Avoid creamy sauces on pasta, meat and fish dishes.
- Choose new potatoes, jacket potatoes, rice or pasta over chips, but if you must have some, share a portion.
- Good choices for main meals include pasta with a tomato-based sauce; a small peppered steak with salad; poached, baked or grilled fish with veg and new potatoes; or chicken chow mein.

400 CALS

● **MUSHROOM RISOTTO** (SERVES 4)
Heat 2tsp oil in a large pan. Add 1 spring onion, finely chopped, and 3 garlic cloves, crushed. Cook for five minutes, stirring occasionally. Add 240g/8^1/$_2$oz risotto rice and 150g/5oz celery, chopped. Cook for two minutes. Stir in 90ml/3^1/$_2$floz white wine and 115g/4oz button mushrooms, sliced. Slowly add 1ltr/1^3/$_4$pt hot stock, stirring frequently, until stock is absorbed into rice. Serve with 65g/2^1/$_2$oz Parmesan cheese, grated, parsley and a large salad with fat-free dressing.

● **ROAST VEG AND WHITE FISH**
Slice 1 carrot, 1 celery stick, 1 onion, 1 red and 1 yellow pepper, and 40g/1^1/$_2$oz fennel and arrange in a roasting dish with 1 garlic clove, chopped, 1tsp olive oil and 1tsp herbes de Provence. Cook in a hot oven for 20 minutes, stirring halfway through, until golden and starting to crisp. Grill 75g/3oz cod and sprinkle with 1tsp grated Parmesan. Serve with 40g/1^1/$_2$oz (dry weight) couscous.

● **CHICKEN KEBABS**
Skewer small chunks of 100g/3^1/$_2$oz chicken breast, 1 small onion, 1 red pepper and 1 courgette. Brush with marinade made from 1tbsp lemon juice, 2tsp honey, 1tbsp chopped coriander and black pepper. Grill, brushing with marinade during cooking. Cut 100g/3^1/$_2$oz potato into wedges. Toss in a bag with 1^1/$_2$tsp olive oil, a pinch of salt, ^{1}/$_2$tsp paprika and 1tsp Italian herbs. Cook in a hot oven for 30 minutes. Serve with the kebabs.

650 CALS

These guidelines will help you keep within limits, even when eating out fast-food style.

KFC
● Triple Crunch sandwich without sauce and a side order of coleslaw.
● 6 Hot Wings and corn on the cob.

McDONALD'S
● Hot dog & ketchup with medium fries and a large Diet Coke; or
● Hamburger with a regular vanilla milkshake; or
● 4 Chicken McNuggets, regular fries, a sundae (no topping) and Diet Coke.
TIPS Milkshakes and desserts are high in calories so stick to small ice creams or sundaes without toppings. Flavoured shakes are higher in calories than vanilla. McDonald's has an excellent Interactive Nutrition Counter on its website, which allows you to select your chosen menu, then gives the calorie count. Check it out and plan your meals in advance at www.mcdonalds.co.uk.

PIZZA EXPRESS
● Caesar salad with side order of tonno e fagioli (tuna and beans); or
● Lasagne and fresh fruit salad.
TIPS Most pizzas are surprisingly high in calories. We suggest Neptune (603 calories).
● At Pizza Hut, go for Italian or Edge bases for lower fat. Avoid all stuffed crusts.
● Share a pizza with a friend and halve the calories. Fill up with a large salad.
● Go for honey and mustard salad dressings instead of the creamy options.
● Fresh fruit salad makes a great low-calorie dessert at only 125 calories on average.

'FREE' VEGETABLES AND FRUIT

● **Artichokes, asparagus, beansprouts, broccoli, Brussels sprouts, cabbage, carrots, cauliflower, celeriac, celery, chicory, courgettes, cucumber, lettuce, mushrooms, onions, peppers, radish, runner beans, spinach, spring greens, tomatoes, watercress.**
● **Cranberries, gooseberries, grapefruit, loganberries, redcurrants, rhubarb, watermelon.**

50 CALS

● A piece of fresh fruit.
● 12 Twiglets.
● 5 mini bread sticks (plain).
● 10 fresh cherries.
● 125g pot of low-calorie yoghurt.
● 1 McVitie's Go Ahead Apple & Sultana Slice.

150 CALS

● 125ml/4^1/$_2$floz glass dry white wine with 3 sesame breadsticks.
● 25g/1oz peanuts.
● Kellogg's Nutri-Grain Bar (130 cals).
● 150g pot Ambrosia low-fat rice pudding (129 cals).
● 75g/3oz baked beans on 1 medium slice wholegrain toast.

250 CALS

● 250ml bottle pure fruit smoothie.
● 75g/3oz salad leaves and 1 tomato, sliced, with 4tsp pesto sauce and 1 small wholemeal roll.
● 1 standard Crunchie plus an apple.
● 75g/3oz baked beans on 2 slices medium wholegrain toast and 1 x reduced fat cheese triangle.
● 1 standard Flake, plus 1 low-calorie yoghurt and 7 strawberries.
● **Anytime breakfast crunch** (makes 10 portions): Mix 2tbsp unsweetened orange juice with 1tbsp groundnut oil, 3tbsp maple syrup and 1tbsp soft brown sugar. Use to coat 250g/9oz rolled oats, 45g/1^1/$_2$oz wheatgerm, 50g/2oz chopped pecan nuts, 1tbsp sesame seeds, 1tbsp sunflower seeds and 150g/5oz dried mixed fruit. Divide between two shallow pie dishes. Bake at 170°C/325°F/gas mark 3. Stir twice during cooking. Remove after 30 minutes or so. Lasts for a week. Great with fresh fruit, 3tbsp yoghurt, or 50ml/2floz semi-skimmed milk.

Eat all day
and lose weight!

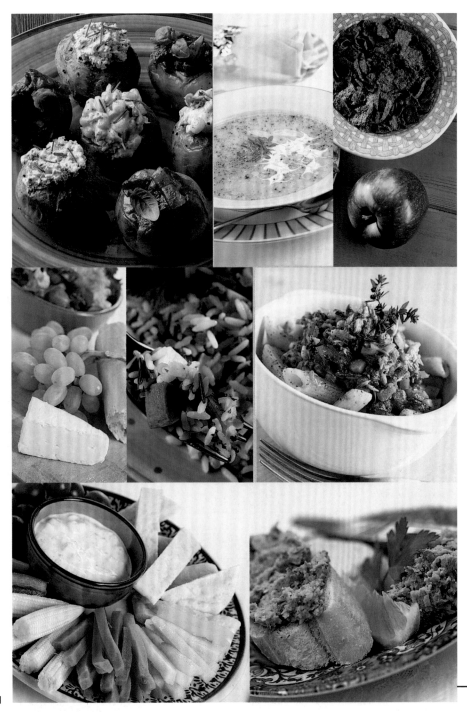

What would you do to get slim?

Cut out a whole food group, never eat carbs and proteins in the same meal, skip lunch for the next six months? There are lots of theories about how to lose fat, few of which produce lasting results. But one theory that does stand up to closer inspection is grazing – spreading your calories across smaller, more frequent meals as a way of keeping your blood sugar levels stable and preventing overeating. Find out how to make grazing work for you – you could drop up to 1st in six weeks!

Eat little and often. Never let yourself get too hungry between each mini meal

6 weeks to a slimmer you!

THE PLAN

Target your weight loss:

Target loss	Cal allowance	Snacks	Plus
Less than 1st	1,350 calories	5	'free' veg
1st to 3st	1,600 calories	6	'free' veg
More than 3st	1,850 calories	7	'free' veg and fat

What to do

● Every day choose 5, 6 or 7 snacks depending on how much you have to lose
● Always have a snack at breakfast
● Don't go for more than two to three hours between eating
● Where menus recommend a certain number of servings check 'How big should portions be?'

Keep it healthy

● At least four of your snacks should come from four different sections each day.
● Each day, have 275ml/¹/₂pt skimmed milk to drink on its own or for tea and coffee. Alternatively, have two pots diet yoghurt or 150ml/¹/₄pt skimmed milk plus one pot diet yoghurt. This is in addition to any milk in the menus. Don't skip this dairy allowance as it provides you with the calcium you need to keep your bones strong and aids weight loss.

● 'Free' veg means you may eat most vegetables (including canned and frozen veg) in unlimited amounts, except for potatoes, sweet potato, yam, parsnips, peas, sweetcorn and beans (French beans and runner beans are OK), which are higher in calories. But don't add any kind of fat to them. Eat your 'free' vegetables as an accompaniment to your snacks or as a snack on their own. You should eat at least five portions of fruit and vegetables every day.
● You can drink unlimited water, black tea and coffee, Bovril, Marmite, low-calorie squashes and fizzy drinks
NB You should aim to lose 1lb-2lb a week, although you may lose more than this at the start, due to water loss as well as fat loss. If you regularly lose more than 2lb a week, you will also be losing muscle.

FEATURE: DELL STANFORD. PHOTOGRAPHY: ANDREW SYDENHAM

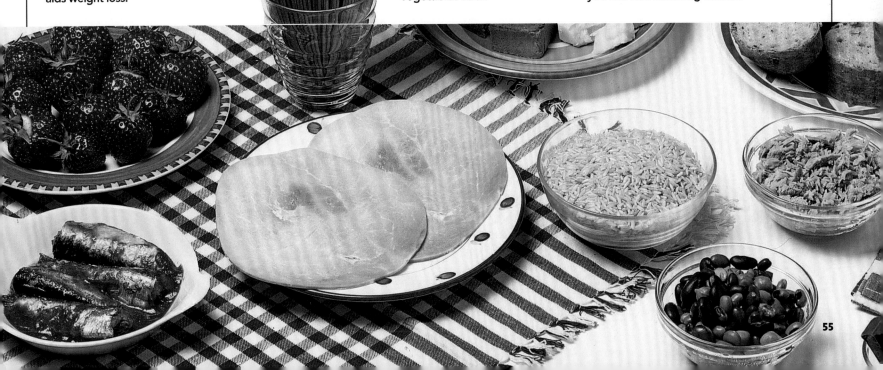

HOW BIG SHOULD PORTIONS BE?

FOOD	SERVING SIZE
Glass unsweetened orange juice	150ml/¼pt
Skimmed milk for cereal	150ml/¼pt
Frozen summer fruit	225g/8oz
Fresh strawberries	175g/6oz
Rice, pasta	40g/1½oz, raw weight
French bread	25g/1oz
Jacket potato, new potatoes	200g/7oz, raw weight
Low-fat oven chips	115g/4oz, raw weight
Low-fat beef burger	50g/2oz, raw weight
Lean skinless chicken breast	150g/5oz, raw weight
Low-fat Brussels pâté, lean ham, lean roast beef	40g/1½oz
Sardines, canned in tomato sauce	75g/3oz
Cod fillet, skinless	115g/4oz, raw weight
Canned mixed beans, drained	50g/2oz
Canned tuna in brine, drained	40g/1½oz
Reduced-fat mozzarella	50g/2oz
Salmon fillet, skinless	75g/3oz, raw weight
Cooked chicken tikka fillets, cooked lean skinless chicken	25g/1oz
Reduced-fat Cheddar cheese	20g/¾oz
Milk chocolate	40g/1½oz

7 good reasons to graze

● Controlling your appetite with regular snacks helps to stop you overeating.

● Eating small, regular meals keeps your metabolism boosted.

● Going for long periods between meals can lower blood sugar levels, leading to tiredness and cravings for high-fat, high-sugar foods.

● Snacks don't have to be unhealthy. In fact, it's often easier to eat the right balance of foods with healthy snacks. You should concentrate on starchy carbohydrate-rich snacks with plenty of fruit and vegetables.

● Snacks are easy to prepare, so you spend less time in the kitchen, which means less temptation to nibble.

● Uncooked food can be just as nutritious as a hot meal. In fact, cooked foods tend to lose more nutrients because not only can heat destroy the nutrients but they also seep out into the cooking water. So eating lots of uncooked snacks can boost your nutrient intake.

● Snacks are portable, so they will fit into your lifestyle.

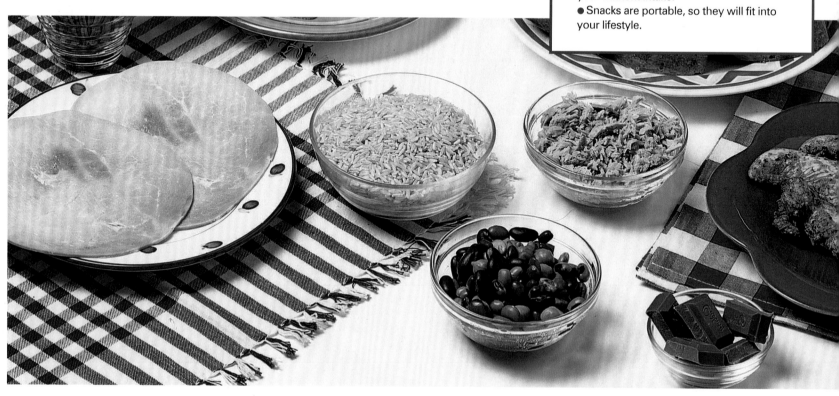

EAT ALL DAY SNACKS (250 calories each)

Wake up to cereal

- 2 wholewheat cereal biscuits with milk and 3 chopped dried apricots.
- 4tbsp bran cereal with milk and 1 small chopped banana.
- 6tbsp cornflakes with milk. Plus 1 pot diet yoghurt.
- 2tbsp unsweetened muesli with milk. Plus 1 glass orange juice.
- 3tbsp porridge oats heated with milk and 1tsp honey. Plus 1 glass orange juice.
- 2tbsp unsweetened muesli mixed with 1 pot low-fat plain yoghurt and 3 chopped apricots.

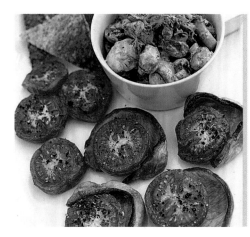

Breakfast bites

- 1 bread roll with 2 grilled lean rashers back bacon, 1 sliced tomato and shredded lettuce.
- 1 boiled or poached egg with 1 slice toast and 1tsp low-fat spread and 1 glass orange juice.
- 2 slices toast with 2tsp low-fat spread and 3tsp jam or marmalade.
- 1 low-fat pork sausage with 150g can baked beans in tomato sauce.
- Make a quick and easy omelette with 2tsp oil and 2 eggs plus 10 sliced closed cup poached mushrooms.
- 1 slice toast with 1tbsp peanut butter and 1 glass orange juice.

- All slices of bread should be medium-sized and rolls should be small. Choose wholemeal, granary, brown or high-fibre white varieties to fill you up.
- Go for wholemeal varieties of pasta and brown or wholegrain rice as they are higher in filling fibre.
- Choose extra-lean meat, remove any visible fat and take the skin off chicken before cooking.
- All pots of yoghurt should be small: 125g or 150g.
- All eggs should be medium-sized.
- All tablespoon and teaspoon measurements should be level: 1tsp=5ml and 1tbsp=15ml.

Pick-a-pitta

1 wholemeal pitta bread with one of the following and salad:
- 2tbsp reduced-cal coleslaw.
- 1 serving reduced-fat cheese.
- 1tbsp low-fat cottage cheese with 1 sliced pineapple ring, canned in natural juice.
- 1 serving canned tuna in brine, drained, with 1tbsp low-fat plain yoghurt.
- 1 serving chicken tikka fillets with 1tbsp low-fat plain yoghurt.
- 1 serving canned mixed beans, drained, plus fat-free vinaigrette.

Baked potatoes

Bake 1 serving potato and serve with one of the following toppings plus 'free' veg:
- 2tbsp canned sweetcorn, with 1tbsp low-fat plain yoghurt.
- 1 serving lean cooked chicken mixed with 1tbsp reduced-calorie mayonnaise and $\frac{1}{2}$tsp mild curry powder.
- $\frac{1}{2}$ x 205g can baked beans in tomato sauce.
- 2tbsp low-fat cottage cheese and 1 sliced tomato.
- $\frac{1}{2}$ x 390g can Ratatouille Provençale.
- 1tbsp reduced-fat houmous.

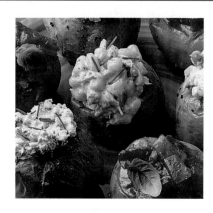

Get fruity

- 1 small banana chopped with 4 crushed walnut halves, 3tbsp low-fat plain yoghurt and 1tsp runny honey.
- 1 serving strawberries with 1 fruit scone and 1tbsp spray cream.
- Make a fruit salad with 1 sliced kiwi, 1 segmented orange, 1 sliced apple, 1 nectarine mixed with 5tbsp unsweetened orange juice.
- Blend together 1 small banana, 1 serving strawberries, 1 pot diet strawberry yoghurt and 150ml/¼pt skimmed milk.
- 1 serving defrosted frozen summer fruit with 1 scoop vanilla ice cream and 2 wafers.
- Mix together the following dried ready-to-eat fruits: 3 dates, 3 apricots, 2tbsp raisins and 1 fig.

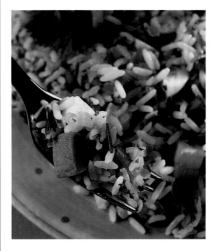

Rice, pasta and potatoes

- 1 serving rice with 1 serving lean cooked chicken, 1tbsp canned sweetcorn, ½ diced red pepper and fat-free vinaigrette.
- 1 serving pasta with ½tbsp pesto sauce.
- Mix 1 serving pasta with 1 serving canned tuna in brine, drained, ½ x 400g can chopped tomatoes, 1tsp chopped fresh herbs and 1tbsp grated parmesan. Heat and serve.
- 1 serving new potatoes, boiled and mixed with 3 sliced spring onions, 1tsp chopped fresh chives, ½ diced red pepper, 1tbsp reduced-calorie mayonnaise and 1tbsp low-fat plain yoghurt.
- Cut 1 serving potato into eight wedges, brush with 1tsp olive oil and bake in a hot oven for 15 minutes. Sprinkle with 1 serving reduced-fat Cheddar cheese.
- 1 serving rice with 3tbsp cooked frozen mixed vegetables, 5 whole cashew nuts and fat-free vinaigrette.

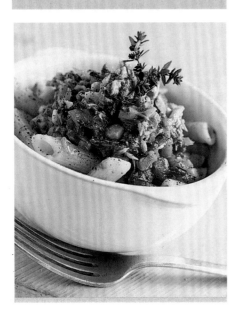

Meat and fish

- **1 serving salmon fillet, grilled, plus 1 serving French bread and 'free' vegetables.**
- **1 serving chicken breast fillet, grilled, plus 1 serving French bread plus 'free' vegetables.**
- **1 bread roll with 2 grilled fish fingers and salad.**
- **1 bread roll with 1 serving low-fat beefburger, grilled, shredded lettuce, 1 sliced tomato and 1tbsp tomato ketchup.**
- **1 serving low-fat oven chips plus 1 serving cod fillet, grilled. Plus 'free' vegetables.**
- **1 serving sardines, canned in tomato sauce, with 1 slice toast and 1 tsp low-fat spread.**

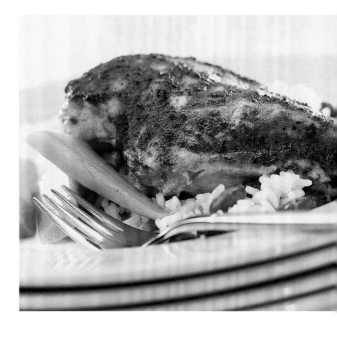

Bready bits
- 1 teacake with 3tsp low-fat spread.
- 1 roll with 1tsp low-fat spread, one of the following fillings and salad:
- 1 sliced hard-boiled egg.
- 1 serving reduced-fat mozzarella cheese and 1 sliced tomato.
- 1 serving low-fat Brussels pâté.
- 1 serving lean ham plus 1 serving reduced-fat Cheddar cheese, grated.
- 1 serving roast beef and mustard.

Sweet treats (twice a week only)
- 2 chocolate mini rolls.
- 3 digestive biscuits.
- 2 scoops chocolate ice cream plus 1 ice cream wafer.
- 1 custard doughnut.
- 1 serving milk chocolate.
- 150g pot custard-style yoghurt.

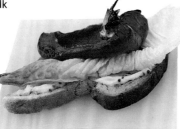

ALCOHOL AND DRINKS

Limit alcohol to twice a week, as it gives calories without many nutrients
- 1 alcoholic drink (see list below) plus one 25g packet low-fat crisps.
- 2 alcoholic drinks (see list below).
- Diet soft drink and 50g pack peanuts and raisins.
- Diet soft drink and 1 regular portion 'fast food' French fries.
- Diet soft drink and 3 slices garlic bread.

One alcoholic drink can be 1 regular glass of wine, 1/2pt normal strength bitter, lager or cider or 2 pub measures of spirit with diet mixer.

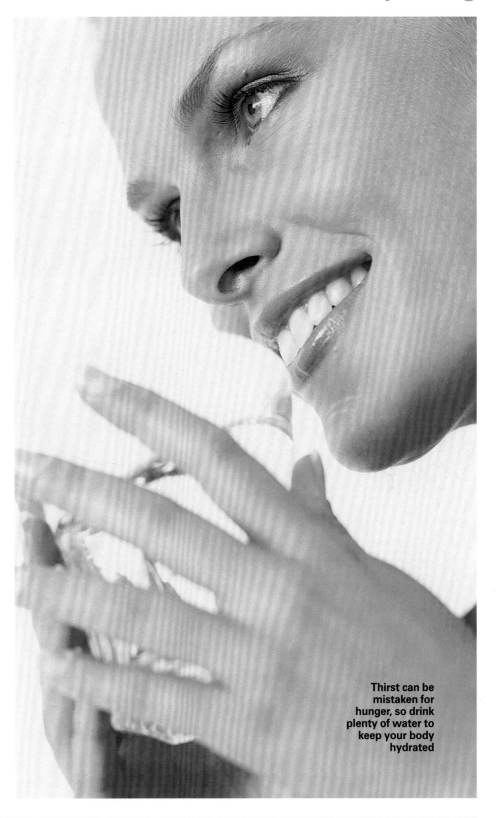

Thirst can be mistaken for hunger, so drink plenty of water to keep your body hydrated

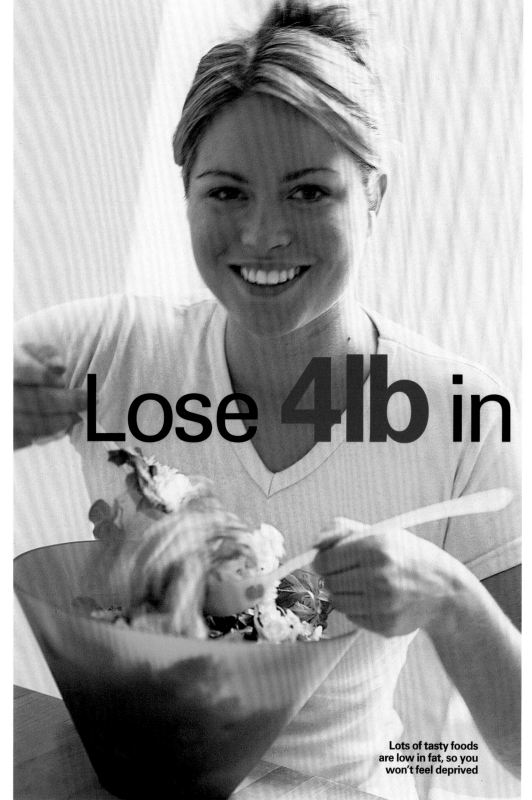

If you eat less fat, you'll lose weight – it's as simple as that. Follow our no-nonsense fat-counting plan and you'll see results in just seven days

Lose 4lb in 7 days

Not everybody likes counting calories but you can't get away from the fact that you have to take in fewer calories than your body needs if you're going to lose weight.

As fatty foods are the most concentrated in calories (with alcohol coming in a fairly close second), it makes sense to eat less of them if you want to lose weight.

So, if you like the idea of counting fat grams rather than calories, this diet is the one for you. We've made the plan as varied as possible, but if you're aiming to lose up to 4lb over the week you're following this diet, you'll need to stick to it rigidly.

If you can, push your energy output up as well, by just being more physically active in your movements – walk faster or further – or actually do some exercise. Not only will it aid your weight loss but it could also help you firm up your body. It's just for seven days, so go for it!

Lots of tasty foods are low in fat, so you won't feel deprived

FEATURE: JANE GRIFFIN. PHOTOGRAPHY: ANDREW SYDENHAM

Read this first!

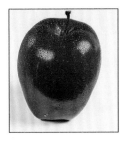

Getting down to basics

Every day you must have one breakfast, one light meal and one main meal and you can also include one snack a day. You can eat your light meal and main meal whenever it suits you but you might like to have your snack after any exercise you do. If you don't need a snack, don't have it – it could tip the scales even more in your favour.

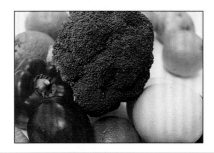

Remember the famous five

When you're planning which of the meals to have, remember that for good health, you should be having five portions of fruit and vegetables every day.

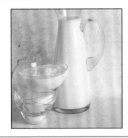

Look after your bones

You need to keep up your calcium intake, so every day have 275ml/$\frac{1}{2}$pt skimmed milk in addition to the milk already in the meals. If you prefer, you may have two small pots of diet yoghurt instead.

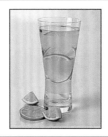

Don't dehydrate

Drink plenty of fluids – water, tea, coffee, herbal teas, Bovril, Marmite and diet or low-calorie soft drinks.

You can still have your fill

You can eat unlimited amounts of vegetables – raw or lightly cooked (boiled, microwaved or steamed) with all light and main meals. Choose from artichokes, asparagus, aubergines, bean sprouts, broccoli, Brussels sprouts, cabbage, carrots, cauliflower, celery, chicory, courgettes, cucumber, fennel, garlic, gherkins, green beans, leeks, lettuce, mangetout, marrow, mushrooms, onions, peppers, pumpkins, radish, spinach, spring greens, swede, tomatoes, turnip and watercress. You can also add herbs (fresh or dried) or spices to any meals.

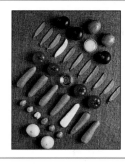

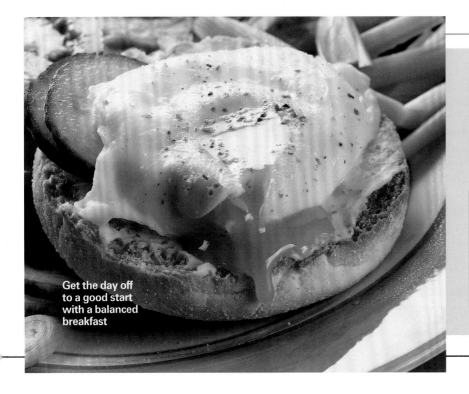

Get the day off to a good start with a balanced breakfast

Breakfasts

(5g fat and around 300 calories)

All recipes serve 1

Hasty breakfast

- 1 small glass unsweetened orange or grapefruit juice
- 1 Jordan's Apricot and Almond Frusli bar
- 1 Müllerlight yoghurt (any flavour)

Savoury breakfast
- 1 plain bagel
- 2tbsp low-fat soft cheese
- 25g/1oz smoked salmon pieces (vegetarian: 1tsp chopped mixed nuts sprinkled on top of the cheese)

Cooked breakfast
- 2 back bacon rashers, trimmed of fat and grilled (vegetarian: 1 medium boiled egg)
- 2 slices medium sliced white bread
- 1tbsp ketchup, spread on bread (vegetarian – omit)
- 1 small glass unsweetened orange or grapefruit juice

Fruit breakfast
- 2 slices medium wholemeal toast
- 2tsp low-fat spread
- 1 small banana, sliced on top of the toast and sprinkled with cinnamon (optional)
- 1 small glass unsweetened orange or grapefruit juice

Breakfast in a bowl
- 150ml/¼pt skimmed milk
- 40g/1½oz bran flakes
- 1tbsp raisins
- 2tsp pumpkin seeds

Light meals
(10g fat and around 350 calories)

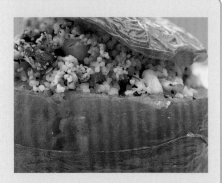

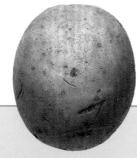

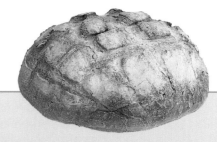

Couscous
- 40g/1½oz couscous, raw weight (prepared according to the instructions on the packet)
- 1 small apple, cored and diced
- 1tbsp sultanas
- 2 heaped tbsp canned red kidney beans, drained

Toss all ingredients in a dressing of 1tbsp olive oil, lemon juice, crushed garlic and herbs of choice.

Jacket potato with beans
- 1 medium jacket potato
- 2tsp low-fat spread
- 150g/5oz can baked beans
- 115g/½oz grated reduced-fat Cheddar cheese

Tuna nicoise salad
- 150g/5oz new potatoes, boiled
- Cooked French beans
- Chopped tomatoes
- 1 hard-boiled egg, cut into wedges
- 1 small can (100g/3½oz) tuna in brine/spring water, drained and flaked

Toss ingredients in a dressing of vinegar, mustard and lemon juice and serve on a bed of salad leaves.
- Plus 1 pot Boots Shapers Strawberry Yoghurt Mousse
- **Vegetarian alternative:** replace tuna with 2tbsp canned sweetcorn

Turkey sandwich
- 2 medium slices wholemeal bread
- 2tsp low-fat spread
- 50g/2oz wafer-thin turkey slices
- 1tbsp cranberry sauce
- 1 medium peach
- **Vegetarian alternative:** 50g/2oz low-fat soft cheese and 3 dried dates

Cheese melt
- 2 medium slices of French bread
- 1 peeled garlic clove, halved
- 1tsp olive oil
- 50g/2oz reduced-fat mozzarella
- Cherry tomatoes

Toast the bread then rub with the garlic and drizzle with oil. Place the mozzarella slices on top and grill until the cheese starts to melt. Serve with cherry tomatoes.

All recipes serve 1

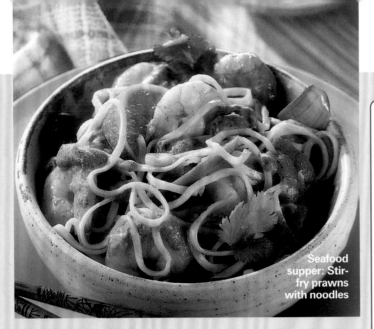

Seafood supper: Stir-fry prawns with noodles

Main meals
(15g fat and around 400 calories)

All recipes serve 1

Stuffed peppers
- 2 large red or yellow peppers, deseeded
- 1tsp vegetable oil
- 1 small onion, chopped
- 1 garlic clove, crushed
- 25g/1oz cooked brown rice
- 25g/1oz raisins
- 25g/1oz mushrooms, chopped
- 6 blanched almonds, chopped
- 1 skinned tomato, chopped
- 1tsp tomato purée

Preheat the oven to 190°C/375°F/gas mark 5. Slice the tops off the peppers and set aside. Blanch the peppers in boiling water for 3 minutes, drain and arrange in a dish. Heat the oil in a pan and add the onion and garlic. Cook until softened, mix in the remaining ingredients. Spoon into the peppers, replace the tops and bake for 30 minutes. Serve.
- Plus 125g/4½oz any low-fat yoghurt

Salmon in a parcel with rice
- 115g/4oz skinless salmon steak
- ½ clove of garlic, sliced
- 1 spring onion, sliced
- 2tsp fresh coriander, chopped
- 2tsp fresh lemon juice
- 115g/4oz boiled or steamed rice
- Any 'free' vegetables of your choice

Preheat the oven to 240°C/475°F/gas mark 9. Cut a piece of foil large enough to make a parcel for the fish. Place the fish on the foil and add the garlic, onion, coriander and lemon juice. Wrap up the parcel and cook for 10 minutes or until the fish is cooked. Boil, steam or microwave the vegetables and serve with the rice and salmon parcel.
- Plus 170g St Ivel Shape Bio Twinpot Yoghurt

Stir-fry prawns with noodles
- 2tsp sunflower oil
- Crushed garlic to taste
- 75g/3oz shelled prawns
- Assorted vegetables eg beansprouts, mangetout
- 1tbsp soy sauce
- 1tbsp low-fat plain yoghurt
- 115g/4oz boiled or steamed noodles
- Chinese Five Spice powder to taste (optional)

Heat the oil in a wok or frying pan and cook the garlic. Add the prawns and stir-fry for 4 minutes. Add the vegetables and soy sauce and stir-fry until the fish is cooked and the vegetables are still crunchy. Stir in the yoghurt and serve with noodles. Add Five Spice powder if desired.
Vegetarian alternative: 115g/4oz tofu
- Plus fresh melon cut into chunks and served with 3tbsp Greek yoghurt

Sausage ragout
- 1tsp sunflower oil
- 1 onion, finely chopped
- 1 yellow pepper, sliced
- ½tsp fennel seeds
- 200g canned tomatoes
- 2 low-fat sausages, grilled
- 115g/4oz cooked pasta

Heat the oil and cook the onion until soft. Add the peppers and cook for 2-3 minutes. Add the fennel seeds and tomatoes and bring to the boil. Simmer the sauce until thickened. Slice the sausages and add to the sauce. Serve with pasta.

Quick burger meal
- 1 medium reduced-fat beefburger, grilled
- 1 small burger bun
- 1 packet lightly salted baked potato crisps
- Large mixed salad
- Dressing: 2tsp olive oil, lemon juice and seasoning to taste
Vegetarian alternative: 1 Southern-style Quorn burger
- Plus dessert bowl of fresh fruit salad

Vegetable macaroni
- 15g/½oz low-fat spread
- 15g/½oz flour
- 150ml/¼pt skimmed milk
- 115g/4oz cooked macaroni
- 225g/8oz cooked carrots, broccoli and peas
- 25g/1oz reduced-fat cheese

Make a sauce with the spread, flour and milk. Add the macaroni and vegetables and stir until coated with the sauce. Tip into a heatproof dish, sprinkle with cheese and grill until the cheese melts.

Roast dinner
- 75g/3oz lean roast pork
- 2tbsp apple sauce
- 4 small boiled potatoes
- 1tsp low-fat spread
- Any 'free' vegetables of your choice
- 3 crispbreads/rice crackers
- 25g/1oz reduced-fat Edam
- Celery sticks
Vegetarian alternative: 150g/5oz Quorn fillets in white wine and mushroom sauce

50-calorie snacks
- 2 sticks celery, 1 medium carrot and 2tbsp low-fat natural yoghurt flavoured with mild curry powder
- 1 carton low-fat fruit yoghurt
- 150ml/¼pt unsweetened fruit juice
- 1 medium piece of fruit
- 150ml/¼pt skimmed milk and a dash of low-sugar Ribena cordial
- 2tbsp raisins
- 3 bread sticks
- 1 Jaffa cake

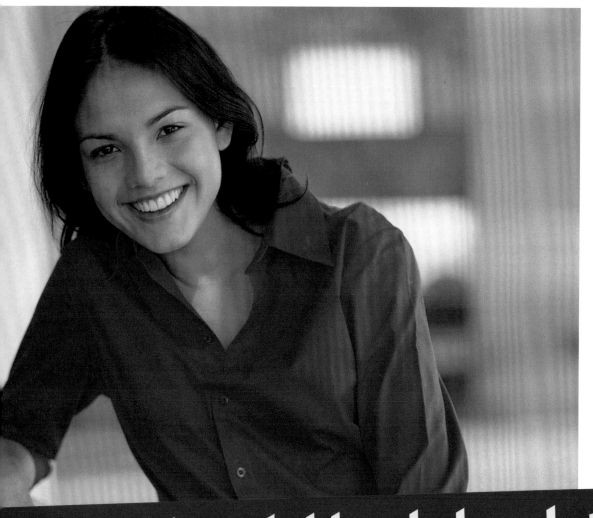

If you follow this diet, you can expect to shift between 1lb and 2lb a week. But it's not unusual to shift more weight in the first week as you lose water as well as fat. So stick to it and you could achieve a total weight loss of 10lb!

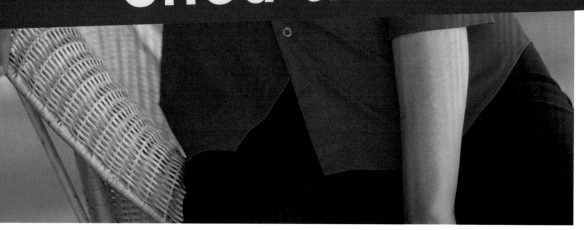

Shed that last 10lbs!

GET ACTIVE

By doing some kind of exercise, you'll build muscle as you lose fat, as muscle needs more calories than fat to function. Plus, you'll burn more calories even when you're not moving around – that means extra weight loss.

Here's what to do

✓ Each day, choose one breakfast, one light meal, one main meal and one, two or three snacks depending on how much you've got to lose (see *How many cals do I need?*). Eat your meals at any time, but try to eat regularly so you don't get hungry.

✓ Every day you should have 275ml/½pt skimmed milk for tea and coffee or just on its own, for essential calcium. This is on top of any milk that appears in the diet itself. If you prefer, you may have two 125g pots of diet yoghurt (any flavour) instead.

✓ Fill up on vegetables, which are low in fat and calories but are packed with vitamins and minerals. It's virtually impossible to eat so many vegetables that you significantly increase your calorie intake, so eat unlimited amounts of

the following, but don't add extra fat or oil: asparagus, aubergines, bean sprouts, broccoli, Brussels sprouts, cabbage, carrots, cauliflower, cucumber, celery, courgettes, garlic, gherkins, green beans, leeks, lettuce, mangetout, marrow, mushrooms, onions, peppers, pumpkins, radish, spinach, spring greens, swede, tomatoes and watercress.

✓ You may drink unlimited amounts of tea and coffee (with sweetener and milk from your allowance). You can also drink unlimited amounts of 'diet' squashes and fizzy drinks, water, yeast or beef extract drinks.

✓ If you have more than 1st to lose you can choose alcohol from the snacks list – but aim to limit this to once or twice a week. If you have less than 1st to lose, alcohol is out for the time being.

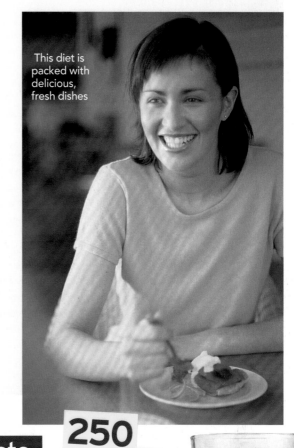

This diet is packed with delicious, fresh dishes

HOW MANY CALS DO I NEED?

GOAL	DAILY CALS	WHAT TO EAT
1ST OR LESS TO LOSE	1,250*	Your three meals, milk allowance, plus one 250-calorie snack
BETWEEN 1ST AND 3ST TO LOSE	1,500*	Your three meals, milk allowance, plus two 250-calorie snacks
MORE THAN 3ST TO LOSE	1,750*	Your three meals, milk allowance, plus three 250-calorie snacks

* Men should add an extra 250 calories to the above figures.

Breakfasts 250 cals

■ **FRUIT LOAF AND JUICE**
Serve 50g/2oz fruit loaf with 2tsp low-fat spread and 150ml/¼pt unsweetened orange juice.

■ **BANANA SHAKE**
Place 1 sliced banana, 1 x 125g pot diet strawberry yoghurt, 50g/2oz strawberries and 150ml/¼pt skimmed milk in a food processor and blend. Chill before serving.

■ **PINEAPPLE MUESLI**
Mix 40g/1½oz unsweetened muesli with 75g/3oz fresh pineapple chunks. Serve with 150ml/¼pt skimmed milk.

■ **CEREAL AND JUICE**
Serve 2 wholewheat cereal biscuits with 150ml/¼pt skimmed milk. Serve with 150ml/¼pt unsweetened orange juice.

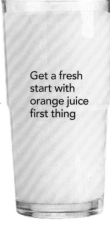

Get a fresh start with orange juice first thing

■ **HONEY MUFFIN**
Split and toast 1 English muffin and top with 2tsp low-fat spread and 1tsp honey.

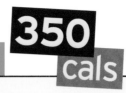

■ PRAWN SANDWICH

Make a sandwich with 2 medium slices wholemeal bread, 40g/1½oz reduced-fat soft cheese, 50g/2oz prawns, peeled, ¼ small apple, diced, and ½ stick celery, sliced. Serve with salad from the unlimited items list.

■ TUNA AND CHEESE BAKED POTATO

Bake a 200g/7oz potato (raw weight) and top with 50g/2oz tuna and 115g/4oz cottage cheese. Serve with salad from the unlimited items list.

■ EASY CHICKEN SALAD

Make a dressing with 2tbsp plain low-fat natural yoghurt, 1tbsp wine vinegar and 1 garlic clove, crushed. Arrange 1 apple, 1 pear and 1 kiwi fruit, all sliced, and 1 orange segment on a plate. Add some lettuce and top with 50g/2oz lean chicken breast, cooked and sliced. Drizzle over the dressing and serve.

■ ENERGY-BOOSTING BEAN SALAD

Mix ½ x 400g can mixed bean salad with 2 spring onions, 1 tomato, 15g/½oz sultanas, ½ stick celery and 50g/2oz plain low-fat yoghurt. Serve with salad from the unlimited items list, opposite. Plus 1 orange.

■ MEDITERRANEAN SALAD

Make a salad from 50g/2oz reduced-fat mozzarella cheese, ¼ red pepper, 1 tomato, lettuce, 5 black olives and 2tbsp fat-free dressing. Serve with 40g/1½oz French bread.

■ POWER PITTA

Fill 1 medium wholemeal pitta bread with 40g/1½oz houmous and salad from the unlimited items list.

■ CHEESY COD WITH RICE

Place a 150g/5oz cod fillet (raw weight) on foil and top with ½ x 400g can chopped tomatoes with herbs and 2 spring onions. Season, seal the foil and place in a medium oven for 20 minutes. Turn out onto a plate and sprinkle with 25g/1oz reduced-fat Cheddar cheese, grated. Place under a hot grill for one minute. Serve with 35g/1¼oz rice (raw weight), boiled, and vegetables from the unlimited items list.

■ GRILLED LAMB

Grill a 115g/4oz lean lamb chop. Boil 115g/4oz spring greens for a few minutes, drain, chop and mix with 1tsp low-fat spread and pepper. Serve with 200g/7oz potatoes, boiled, 6tbsp fat-free gravy and vegetables from the unlimited items list.

■ EASY MUSHROOM RISOTTO

Heat 1tsp oil in a non-stick pan. Chop 1 small onion and crush 1 garlic clove. Add to the pan and cook until soft. Add 75g/3oz mushrooms, sliced, 50g/2oz risotto rice (raw weight) and cook for a few minutes. Slowly add 150ml/¼pt vegetable stock. Simmer until the risotto is creamy, add a pinch of nutmeg and season. Serve with salad from the unlimited items list. Plus 1 apple.

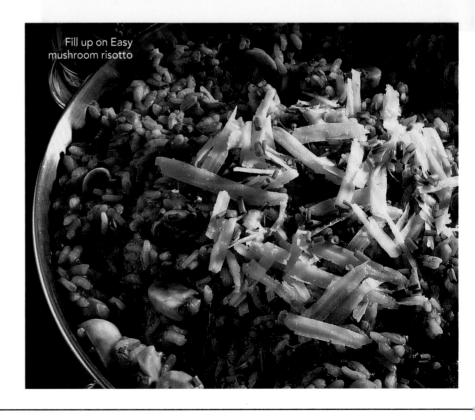

Fill up on Easy mushroom risotto

■ CHICKEN STIR-FRY

Slice 115g/4oz lean skinless chicken breast and stir-fry in 1tsp oil with 1 garlic clove, crushed, for three minutes. Add 2 spring onions, sliced, and 50g/2oz mushrooms, sliced. Cook for two minutes before adding 100g /3½oz rice (raw weight), cooked, 25g/1oz frozen peas, 1tbsp soy sauce and 25g/1oz bean sprouts. Fry for another two minutes. Garnish with fresh parsley.

■ SMOKED TROUT

Serve 115g/4oz skinless smoked trout with veg from the unlimited items list and 40g/1½oz rice (raw weight), boiled.

■ TOMATO CHOWDER

Heat 1tsp oil in a non-stick pan and add ½ onion and 1 garlic clove, chopped. Sauté for a few minutes. Add 275g/10oz potato (raw weight), diced, a 400g can chopped tomatoes, ½ green pepper and 2tsp chilli sauce. Mix and simmer for 20 minutes.

■ GARLIC MUSHROOMS

Heat 1tsp oil in a non-stick pan. Sauté 1 garlic clove, crushed, and 115g/4oz mushrooms. Stir in 25g/1oz reduced-fat soft cheese with herbs. Bake a 275g/10oz potato (raw weight) and top with mushrooms. Serve with salad from the unlimited items list. Plus 1 banana.

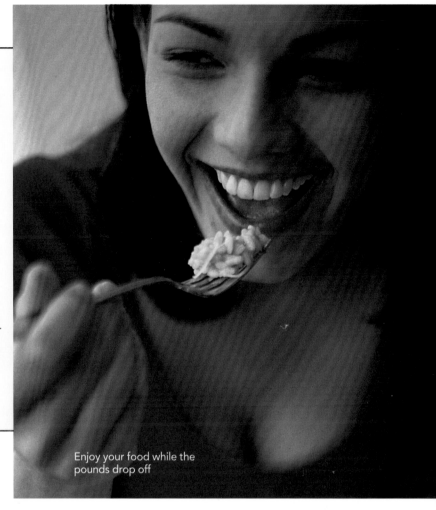

Enjoy your food while the pounds drop off

Snacks 250 cals

■ FRUIT SELECTION

Eat the following separately or chopped and mixed together to make a fruit salad: 1 small banana, 1 kiwi fruit, 1 apple, 150g/5oz melon and 150g/5oz pineapple flesh.

■ FRUIT SCONE

Serve 1 scone with 2tsp each of low-fat spread and jam.

■ TOASTED HOT CROSS BUN AND YOGHURT

Toast 1 hot cross bun and top with 2tsp low-fat spread. Plus a 125g pot diet yoghurt.

■ FRUIT AND NUTS

50g bag of mixed nuts and raisins.

■ BLT SANDWICH

Grill 2 rashers of lean back bacon and serve in 2 medium slices wholemeal bread with 1 sliced tomato and some shredded lettuce.

■ BAKED BEANS ON TOAST

Toast 1 medium slice wholemeal bread and top with 1tsp low-fat spread and a 205g can baked beans in tomato sauce.

■ HOT CHOCOLATE AND BISCUITS

2 chocolate digestive biscuits, plus 2 mugs hot chocolate made with two sachets reduced-calorie hot chocolate drink. Limit this treat to twice a week.

■ ICE CREAM

150g/5oz ice cream. Limit this treat to once a week.

■ CHOCOLATE BAR

50g/2oz bar chocolate. You should limit this treat to twice a week.

■ ALCOHOL AND CRISPS

275ml/½pt normal strength lager, bitter or cider OR 2 pub measures of a spirit with a diet mixer OR a 150ml/5floz glass wine. Plus 1 small packet of crisps. Limit this treat to twice a week.

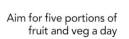

Aim for five portions of fruit and veg a day

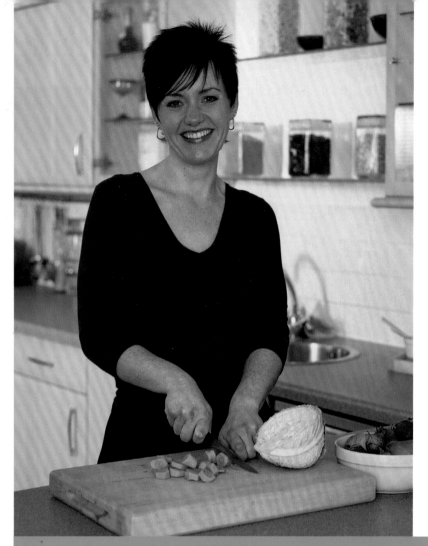

PHOTOGRAPHY: SIMON SMITH. FOOD STYLING: SALLY MANSFIELD

Vanessa Hodkinson became *Slimming Magazine's* 2003 Slimmer of the Year. Want to follow Vanessa's diet plan? Our consultant dietitian Jane Griffin has created an easy diet based on what our winner ate. Vanessa followed a veggie diet, but our diet includes meat. Vanessa had a chocolatey treat each day, and stuck to 1,500 calories a day until she had 3st to lose. She then dropped to 1,250 calories a day, then 1,100 for the last 10lb (but we suggest you up your activity level instead...)

EVERY DAY

■ If you have less than 3st to lose, follow the basic diet of 1,250 calories, which includes: one breakfast, one midday meal, one evening meal and one snack. Have 275ml/½pt skimmed milk for tea, coffee, cereal or on its own. Have two portions of fruit with meals or as a snack.

■ If you have more than 3st to lose, make the basic diet up to 1,500 calories by adding an extra 250 calories from the ideas in the "Do you have more than 3st to lose" box.

The diet that did it!

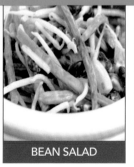

BEAN SALAD

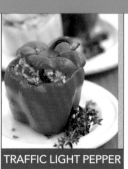

TRAFFIC LIGHT PEPPER

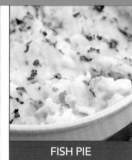

FISH PIE

PLUS:

■ Unlimited amounts of veg – raw or lightly cooked (boiled, steamed or microwaved) with all midday and evening meals. Have three different veg (count a salad as one) during the day and vary what you eat so you don't get bored.

■ Drink plenty of fluids – water, sugar-free squash, tea, coffee, herbal teas, Bovril, Marmite and diet soft drinks.

■ Use lemon juice or 1tbsp fat-free vinaigrette dressing on salads that don't already have one. Choose from any of the following to pep your meals up: freshly ground black pepper, garlic, light soy sauce, Worcestershire sauce, Oriental fish sauce, lemon or lime juice, fresh or dried herbs and spices and sweetener.

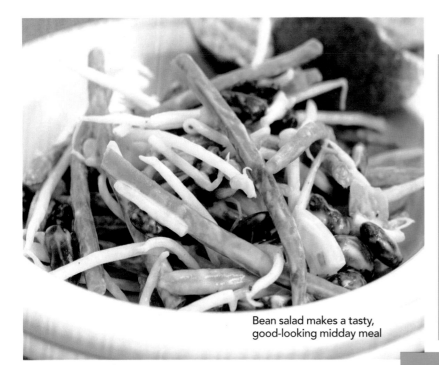

Bean salad makes a tasty, good-looking midday meal

SNACK IDEAS

no more than125 calories

- Bag of Snack-A-Jacks (excluding the caramel variety)
- 30g bag Jacob's Original Twiglets
- 150ml/5fl oz glass of dry or medium wine (red or white)
- 2 pub measures of spirits with low-calorie mixers
- 2-finger Kit Kat
- 1 Marks & Spencer Walnut Whip
- Mr Kipling Apple & Raisin (or Sultana) Flapjack
- Mr Kipling Mini ~~~~~~~
- Cadbury's Chocolate Mini Roll
- Marks & Spencer Count On Us... Trifle
- Marks & Spencer Count On Us... Chocolate Mousse
- Mullerice 99% Fat-Free (150g pot) – Original or Strawberry
- Walls Strawberry Split
- Add your own favourites to the list – just as long as it's within the calorie allowance.

Pile your plate high with vegetables:

Artichokes, asparagus, aubergines, bean sprouts, broccoli, Brussels sprouts, cabbage, carrots, cauliflower, celery, chicory, courgettes, cucumber, fennel, garlic, gherkins, green beans, leeks, lettuce, mangetout, marrow, mushrooms, onions, peppers, pumpkins, radish, spinach, spring greens, swede, tomatoes, turnip and watercress. Peas and sweetcorn are the only veg that Vanessa did not eat in unlimited amounts as they have a higher calorie count than other vegetables.

DO YOU HAVE MORE THAN 3ST TO LOSE?

Make your diet up to 1,500 calories a day with 250 additional calories. Here are some suggestions:

- 1tbsp (40g) cooked rice: 55 calories
- 1tbsp (30g) cooked pasta: 25 calories
- 1 average-sized new potato: 25 calories
- 1 small jacket potato (200g/7oz): 150 calories
- 1 large wholemeal pitta bread: 175 calories
- 1 medium slice wholemeal bread: 75 calories
- 1 crispbread: 30 calories
- 1 large banana: 115 calories
- For breakfast cereals – use the nutritional information on the box

BREAKFASTS `200 cals` All breakfasts serve 1

1 Cereal
Choose from one of the following:
- 2 Weetabix or 2 Shredded Wheats
- 40g/1½oz Wheat or Bran Flakes or Shreddies
- 40g/1½oz Fruit and Fibre cereal
- 3tbsp raw, quick-cook oatmeal served with milk from daily allowance.

Plus 200ml/7fl oz unsweetened orange or grapefruit juice

2 Egg & toast
2 medium slices wholemeal toast, spread with 2tsp low-fat spread, plus 1 boiled egg

3 Toast and marmalade
2 medium slices of wholemeal toast, topped with 2tsp low-fat spread and 2tsp marmalade

4 Cheesy muffin
1 toasted muffin, topped with 2tbsp low-fat soft cheese. Plus 115ml/4fl oz unsweetened orange or grapefruit juice

LUNCHES 300 cals

1 Jacket potato

Serve a 200g/7oz baked potato, uncooked weight, with either 3tbsp baked beans, 50g/2oz low-fat soft cheese or a small can tuna in brine or water. Plus 125g pot virtually fat-free yoghurt. **Serves 1.**

2 Curried parsnip soup

Have one serving of the soup with a wholemeal roll and salad box of unlimited raw veg, plus 125g pot virtually fat-free yoghurt.
Melt 25g/1oz low-fat spread in a pan, stir in 1tsp curry powder and cook for 2 minutes. Add 2 large onions and 575g/1½lb parsnips, peeled and chopped, cook gently for 5 minutes, stirring occasionally. Add 575ml/1pt vegetable stock, season to taste. Bring to the boil, cover and simmer for 25 minutes. Leave to cool then blend. Return soup to pan, add 275ml/½pt skimmed milk and 150ml/¼pt low-fat natural yoghurt. Bring to the boil, stirring. Dice 1 red apple, toss in a little lemon juice and use as a garnish. Season with freshly ground pepper. **Serves 6.**

3 Apple and cheese salad

Have one serving of this salad with 3 crispbreads or 3 rice cakes.
Wash but don't peel 2 juicy eating apples. Core, quarter and cube them. Mix with 2tbsp lemon juice. Add 50g/2oz celery, diced, 50g/2oz raisins, 50g/2oz walnuts, chopped, 100g/3½oz reduced-fat Edam, diced, and mix. Add 4tbsp low-fat natural yoghurt, ¼tsp cinnamon (optional) and a few drops of lemon juice. Mix the salad and yoghurt together. Shred some Chinese leaves, put in salad bowl and spoon the mixture on top. **Serves 4.**

4 Bean salad with yoghurt dressing

Have one serving with 1 mini pitta, plus 125g pot virtually fat-free yoghurt. Mix 175g/6oz fresh or frozen whole green beans, 175g/6oz canned red kidney beans, 175g/6oz

beansprouts,1 small green pepper, chopped, 1 small onion, chopped. Toss veg in a dressing made from 150g pot low-fat natural yoghurt, ¼tsp mustard powder, crushed garlic, 1tsp lemon juice and 1tsp vinegar. Season with freshly ground pepper. Serves 2.

5 Cheesy fruit potatoes

Have one serving, plus 125g pot virtually fat-free yoghurt.
Set oven to 200°C/400°F/gas mark 6. Bake 2 medium potatoes, scrubbed and pricked for 1-1½ hours. Mix together 50g/2oz low-fat natural cottage cheese, 50g/2oz raisins, 50g/2oz dried apricots, chopped and season with freshly ground pepper. Slit the cooked potatoes almost in half and spoon in the filling. Sprinkle with chives. **Serves 2.**

6 Prawn pasta

Have one serving with 2 rice cakes or crispbreads, plus 125g pot virtually fat-free yoghurt. Cook 75g/3oz dried pasta shells as instructions. Drain and rinse under running water; drain again. Mix with 1 apple, cored, sliced and brushed with lemon juice, and 150g/5oz cooked peeled prawns. Blend 4tbsp low-fat natural yoghurt, 3tbsp low-fat natural fromage frais and 1tbsp tomato purée and mix in. **Serves 4.**

7 Bought sandwiches

(APPROX 240 CALS PER PACK)
Have either Marks & Spencer Count On Us… Beef Salad, Chicken No mayonnaise **or** Chinese Chicken Flatbread **or** this DIY option: 2 slices wholemeal bread with a scraping of low-fat spread and: 50g/2oz any lean meat, or small can tuna in brine or water, or 75g/3oz veggie pâté. Serve with a salad box containing unlimited raw veg of choice, plus 125g pot virtually fat-free yoghurt. **Serves 1.**

425 cals
MAIN MEALS

1 Fish & new potatoes

Boil 150g/5oz new potatoes in their skins. Bake 150g/5oz white fish fillet, like cod, with mushrooms, herbs and lemon juice in foil in a medium oven for 20 minutes. Plus 2tbsp peas. **Serves 1.**

2 Stuffed peppers

Have one serving with unlimited veg, plus 2 Mini Babybel Light cheeses and crispbreads or rice cakes.
Set oven to 190°C/375°F/gas mark 5. Slice the tops off 4 x 175g/6oz peppers, and set aside. Discard seeds. Blanche peppers for 3 minutes, drain

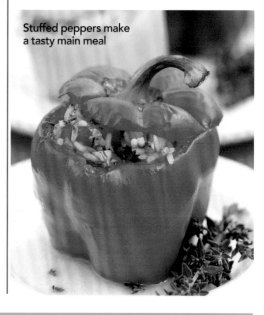

Stuffed peppers make a tasty main meal

WHAT IS A PORTION OF FRUIT?

- ☐ Large slice of melon with ginger (optional)
- ☐ 6 fresh apricots
- ☐ 6 fresh lychees
- ☐ 75g/3oz grapes
- ☐ 150g/5oz fresh cherries
- ☐ Large pear, apple, orange or nectarine
- ☐ Large bowl of raspberries, strawberries, blackberries, gooseberries or rhubarb
- ☐ 6 fresh plums
- ☐ 1 whole grapefruit
- ☐ 2 slices pineapple, fresh or canned in natural juice
- ☐ 1 small banana

and arrange in an ovenproof dish. Heat 1tbsp vegetable oil in a pan and add 1 medium onion, chopped and 1 garlic clove, crushed. Cook until softened, remove from pan and mix with 75g/3oz cooked brown rice, 75g/3oz raisins, 50g/2oz mushrooms, wiped and chopped, 25g/1oz blanched almonds, chopped, 2 tomatoes, skinned and chopped and 1tbsp tomato purée. Divide between peppers, replace tops and bake for 25-30 minutes. **Serves 2.**

3 Fish pie

Have one serving with unlimited veg, plus 50g/2oz lemon sorbet. Set oven to 180°C/ 350°F/gas mark 4. Bake 450g/1lb white fish in a dish with a little water and 1 bay leaf for 20-30 minutes. Drain and remove skin or bones and flake into chunks. Melt 50g/ 2oz low-fat spread in a pan, add 50g/2oz plain flour, mix. Add 575ml/1pt skimmed milk, whisking until thickened. Add 1/2tsp mustard and 100g/31/2oz low-fat Cheddar, grated; stir. Stir in the fish and 100g/31/2oz cooked and peeled prawns. Season with freshly ground black pepper, turn into ovenproof dish. Boil 450g/1lb potatoes, mash with a little low-fat spread and skimmed milk and smother over fish pie. Bake at 180°C/350°F/gas mark 4 for 20 minutes. **Serves 4.**

4 Veggie tagliatelle

Have one serving, plus 1/2 x 225g pot Yeo Valley Fruit Compote with 1tbsp plain yoghurt. Cook 350g/12oz tagliatelle, fresh or dried, according to instructions. Spray a pan with one-calorie spray oil, add 1 medium onion, peeled and chopped, 1 garlic clove, peeled and chopped and cook until softened. Add 3 courgettes, washed and diced, and cook for 5 minutes. Add a 400g can tomatoes, 2tsp fresh basil, chopped, 75g/3oz cooked peas and simmer for 5 minutes. Pour the sauce over the pasta and serve immediately. **Serves 4**

5 Home-made pizza

Have half a Napolina Thin & Crispy Pizza Base, spread with 2tbsp tomato purée topped with a small can chopped, drained tomatoes and 50g/2oz reduced-fat Cheddar, grated. Cook according to directions. Serve with large salad. **Serves 1.**

6 Tandoori chicken

Have one serving with 1 wholemeal pitta and a large salad. Plus 200ml/7fl oz unsweetened orange or grapefruit juice. Preheat oven to 200°C/400°F/ gas mark 6. Remove skin from 8 chicken drumsticks, make 3 slashes in each and rub with lemon juice. Mix 2 garlic cloves, crushed, 1in fresh ginger, grated, 1/2tsp chilli powder, 1/2tsp ground cumin, 1tbsp paprika, 1tbsp garam masala, 1tbsp tomato purée and 150ml/1/4pt low-fat natural yoghurt to form a thick paste. Cover drumsticks with it, place in a roasting tin and roast for about 40 minutes. **Serves 4.**

7 Curried fish

Have one serving with 3tbsp cooked rice and a large salad. Plus 2tbsp plain yoghurt flavoured with low-sugar blackcurrant cordial. Peel 450g/1lb potatoes, cut into even-size cubes and parboil for 5 minutes. Heat 1tbsp sunflower oil in a large pan and cook 1 medium onion, chopped, for 5 minutes. Add 2 garlic cloves, crushed, 15g/1/2oz fresh ginger root, crushed, 1/2tsp turmeric, 1tsp chilli powder, 1tsp ground cumin, 1tsp ground coriander, and 1tsp garam masala. Cook for 1 minute. Add 450g/1lb white fish fillet, skinned and cut into 1in pieces, 1 green pepper and 1 small red pepper, seeded and sliced, the potatoes and 400g can chopped tomatoes. Bring to the boil, simmer for 10 minutes. **Serves 4.**

8 Chicken goulash

Have one serving with 150g/ 5oz cooked egg noodles, plus large green salad. Preheat oven to 160°C/325°F/ gas mark 3. Mix 25g/1oz plain flour, pinch of mustard powder and 1tbsp paprika and toss 565g/11/4lb boneless chicken, skinned and cubed in flour mix. Heat 2tbsp sunflower oil in a pan; brown the chicken and transfer to casserole. Fry 2 medium onions, sliced, 1 large green and 1 large red pepper, seeded and sliced. Add to casserole with 575ml/1pt veg stock and 400g can chopped tomatoes. Cook in the oven for 1-11/2 hours. Spoon 150ml/ 1/4pt low-fat, natural yoghurt and serve. **Serves 4.**

9 Lamb kebabs

Have one serving with 1 wholemeal pitta bread, warmed. Cut 450g/1lb lean lamb into 11/2in cubes. Mix 5tbsp lemon juice, 5tbsp soy sauce and 1 garlic clove, crushed. Marinate meat in this mixture for at least 2 hours. Thread the meat onto long skewers alternating with 8 cherry tomatoes, 12 button or small mushrooms, trimmed, 1 large green pepper, de-seeded and cut into squares, 1 medium onion cut into wedges. Grill kebabs for 15 minutes, turning and basting with marinade sauce. Heat and serve remaining sauce with kebabs. Mix half a small cabbage, grated, 4 carrots, grated, 2 small apples, cored but not peeled and diced. Serve with kebabs and warmed pitta bread. **Serves 4**

10 Ready meals

(**APPROX 240 CALORIES PER PACK**) eg Marks & Spencer Count On Us... (or Safeway's) Ham & Mushroom Tagliatelle, and unlimited veg. Plus any Safeway Healthy Choice Real Fruit Fool. **Serves 1.**

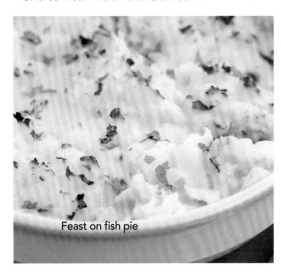

Feast on fish pie

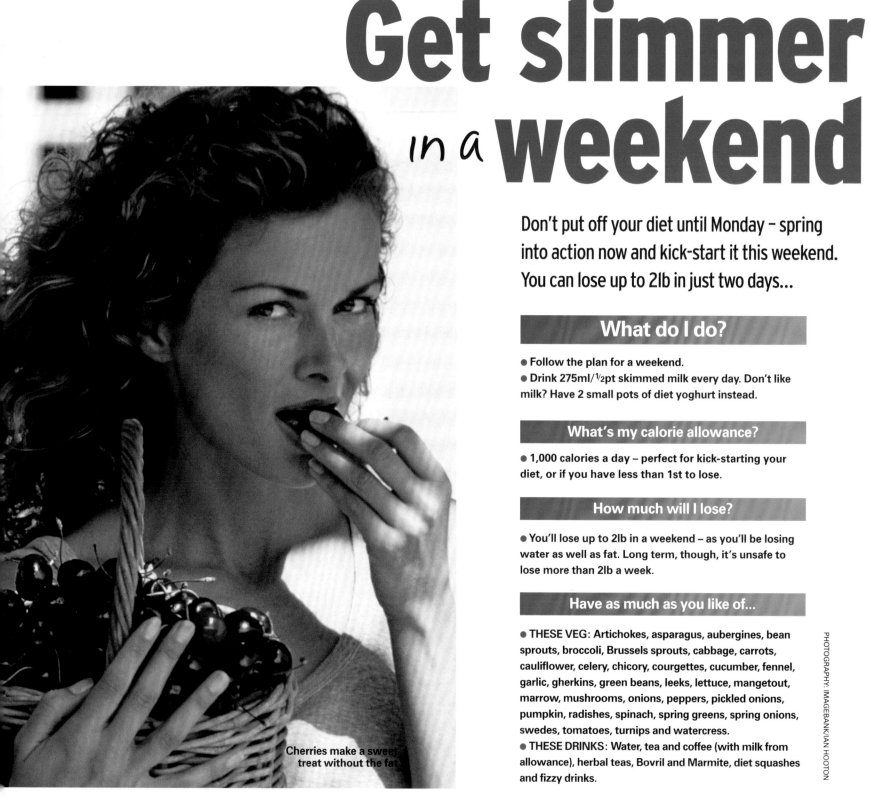

Get slimmer
in a weekend

Don't put off your diet until Monday – spring into action now and kick-start it this weekend. You can lose up to 2lb in just two days...

What do I do?

● Follow the plan for a weekend.
● Drink 275ml/½pt skimmed milk every day. Don't like milk? Have 2 small pots of diet yoghurt instead.

What's my calorie allowance?

● 1,000 calories a day – perfect for kick-starting your diet, or if you have less than 1st to lose.

How much will I lose?

● You'll lose up to 2lb in a weekend – as you'll be losing water as well as fat. Long term, though, it's unsafe to lose more than 2lb a week.

Have as much as you like of...

● THESE VEG: Artichokes, asparagus, aubergines, bean sprouts, broccoli, Brussels sprouts, cabbage, carrots, cauliflower, celery, chicory, courgettes, cucumber, fennel, garlic, gherkins, green beans, leeks, lettuce, mangetout, marrow, mushrooms, onions, peppers, pickled onions, pumpkin, radishes, spinach, spring greens, spring onions, swedes, tomatoes, turnips and watercress.
● THESE DRINKS: Water, tea and coffee (with milk from allowance), herbal teas, Bovril and Marmite, diet squashes and fizzy drinks.

Cherries make a sweet treat without the fat.

Saturday

A light and refreshing way to start the day

Breakfast

SWEET GRAPEFRUIT AND WHOLEMEAL TOAST

Serve ½ grapefruit sprinkled with artificial sweetener and 1 medium slice wholemeal bread, toasted and topped with 5ml/1tsp each of low-fat spread and reduced-sugar jam.

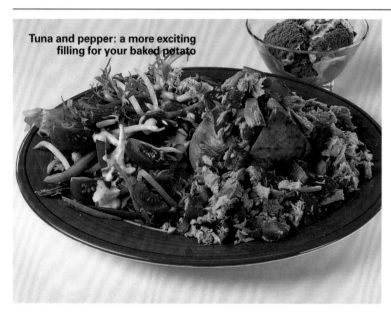

Tuna and pepper: a more exciting filling for your baked potato

Light meal

TUNA AND PEPPER-FILLED BAKED POTATO

Chop ½ green pepper, ½ red pepper and 1 spring onion. Mix with 50g/2oz canned tuna in brine, 50g/2oz red kidney beans and a dash of chilli sauce. Serve with a 200g/7oz jacket potato (raw weight) and unlimited vegetables.

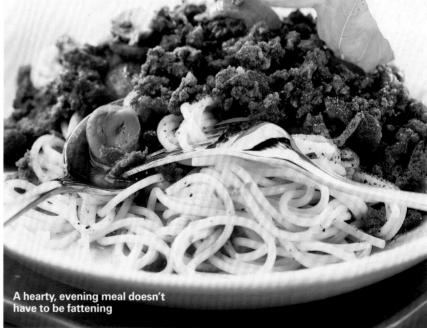

Main meal

SPAGHETTI BOLOGNESE

Finely slice ½ small onion, 1 carrot, 75g/3oz mushrooms and 1 garlic clove. Dry-fry 75g/3oz extra-lean minced beef in a nonstick pan until lightly browned and drain off meat juices. Add the vegetables and garlic to the minced beef. Cook gently until softened. Add 200g can tomatoes, 1tbsp tomato purée, 150ml/¼pt beef stock, 1tbsp mixed herbs and seasonings. Boil and simmer until sauce thickens. Serve with 50g/2oz wholewheat spaghetti (dry weight), boiled, and unlimited salad. Plus 1 kiwi fruit.

A hearty, evening meal doesn't have to be fattening

Sunday

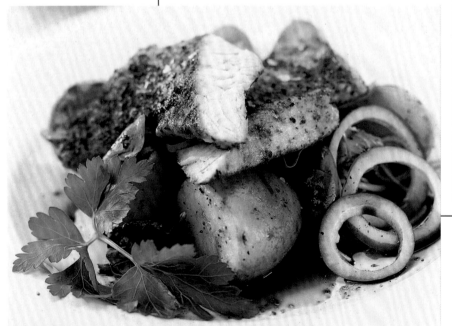

Enjoy this traditional English breakfast, without the fat of frying

Breakfast

COOKED BREAKFAST
Grill 1 lean rasher back bacon, 1 small low-fat sausage, 1 tomato and 5 mushrooms. Serve with 1 medium egg, scrambled with 1tbsp skimmed milk and seasonings.

Light meal

PLOUGHMAN'S LUNCH
Serve 50g/2oz French bread with 40g/1½oz Brie, 15ml/1tbsp pickle. Plus a small bunch of grapes.

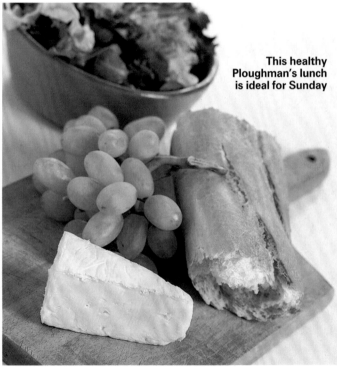

This healthy Ploughman's lunch is ideal for Sunday

Main meal

CHICKEN AND VEGETABLES
Serve 115g/4oz skinless chicken with 4tbsp fat-free gravy, 150g/6oz boiled potatoes and unlimited veg.

Boiled potatoes contain half the calories of roasted ones, so you can have a generous portion

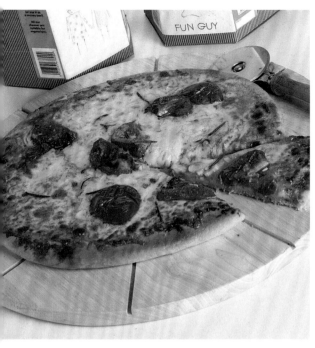

Better by half: you can still enjoy a Saturday-night pizza

Take it away

If you simply *must* have a takeaway at weekends, don't panic. Opt for one of the following in place of your Saturday or Sunday main meal

- 1 portion beef in oyster sauce with ½ portion boiled rice.
- 1 prawn chop suey plus 4 prawn crackers.
- ½ portion chicken and mushrooms with ½ portion special fried rice.
- 1 fish cake plus ½ portion chips.
- 1 portion chicken tikka plus ½ portion boiled rice.
- 1 vegetable curry plus ½ portion boiled rice.
- 2 poppadoms with 1tbsp cucumber raita plus ½ portion jalfrezi and ½ portion boiled rice.
- ½ medium thin-crust pizza.

Boogie nights

Forget about the cinema or sitting in the pub on Saturday night. Instead get your friends together, put on your dancing shoes and bop the night away. Two hours of dancing will burn an amazing 620 calories. But remember to cool down with 'diet' drinks or water rather than alcohol. To help you resist the temptation of an alcoholic tipple, offer to drive. Your friends will love you forever!

A family affair

Plan activities you can do with your family. If the weather's good, go for a walk in the park or the country. One hour of brisk walking will use up to 280 calories. Cycling, even at a leisurely pace, uses up to 140 calories in 30 minutes, while a 30-minute fast swim burns 350 calories. Even floating on your back helps tone your stomach muscles.

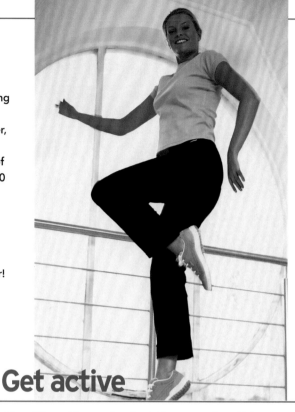

Get active

Spend time at the weekend catching up on chores? Just look how many calories you'll burn off in 10 minutes…

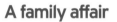

Chore	Calories	Chore	Calories
Vacuuming	45	Ironing	20
Dusting	20	Changing the beds	40
Mowing the lawn	65	Cleaning the windows	40
Polishing the car	40	Mopping the floor	40

Work that body

Sunday mornings are a great time to go to the gym or try an aerobics class because most people are enjoying a lie in. The gym will be really quiet – making it perfect if you feel self-conscious about your body, as there won't be many people around to see you. And when you consider that an hour of low-impact aerobics will burn up to 350 calories, half an hour on the exercise bike will use up 245 calories and 30 minutes on the treadmill burns 315 calories, you'll be able to really enjoy your Sunday roast.

All calorie values stated above are based on a body weight of 11st 1lb.

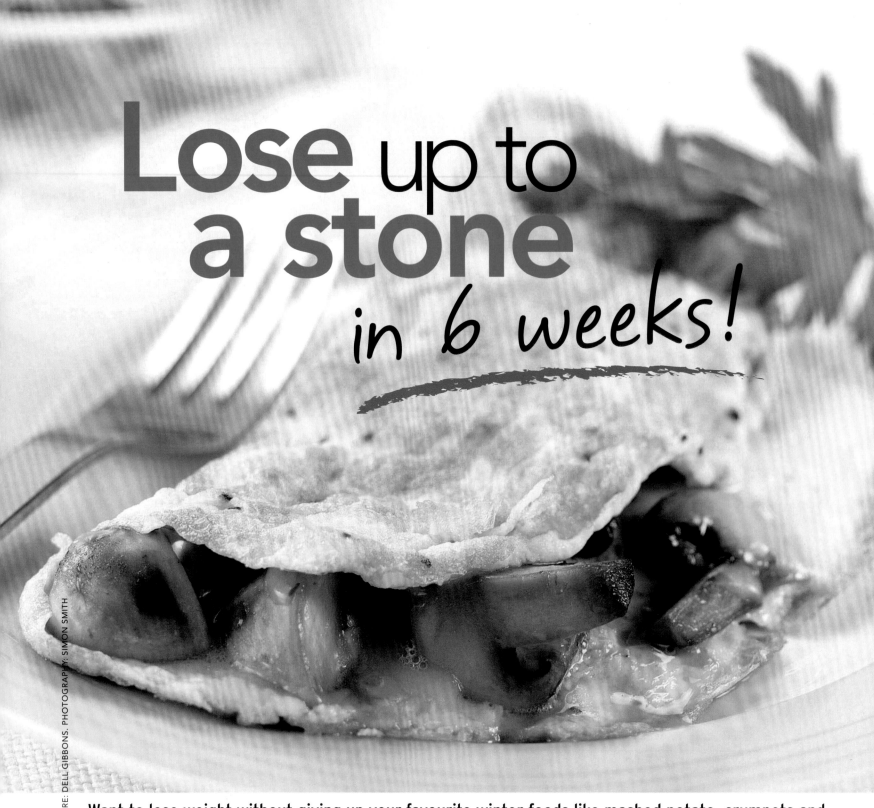

Lose up to a stone in 6 weeks!

FEATURE: DELL GIBBONS. PHOTOGRAPHY: SIMON SMITH

Want to lose weight without giving up your favourite winter foods like mashed potato, crumpets and sticky puddings? This simple diet will satisfy your taste buds, fill you up and blast off pounds, too!

This diet couldn't be easier

Just choose from the recipe options to make a diet plan that suits your lifestyle. If you follow it for six weeks and vary your choices a much as possible you can expect to lose up to 1st.

Step 1: Set your calorie allowance

Your daily calorie allowance will depend on how much weight you want to lose, see below. Each day, choose one breakfast, one light meal and one main meal plus one, two or three snacks, depending on how much you have to lose.

Step 2: Get your five a day

To stay healthy, eat at least five portions of fruit and veg every day, providing you don't cook or serve them with oil, butter, margarine, low-fat spread or oily salad dressings. Choose from: artichokes, asparagus, aubergines, beansprouts, broccoli, Brussels sprouts, cabbage, carrots, cauliflower, celery, chicory, courgettes, cucumber, fennel, garlic, gherkins, green beans, leeks, lettuce, mangetout, marrow, mushrooms, onions, peppers, pumpkins, radish, spinach, spring greens, swede, tomatoes, turnip and watercress. In the meal choices, these are referred to as 'free' vegetables and 'free' salad.

Step 3: Get vital calcium

Don't forget to have $^1/_2$pt of skimmed milk for coffees and teas or drink on its own (this is in addition to any milk that appears in the meals). Or, if you prefer, you can eat two small pots of diet yoghurt instead to get your daily calcium allowance.

To lose	Cals	Breakfast	Light meal	Main meal	Snack(s)
Less than 1st	1,250	1	1	1	1
1st to 3st	1,500	1	1	1	2
More than 3st	1,750	1	1	1	3

All recipes serve 1, unless otherwise stated.

Lose it for keeps!

To lose weight safely and effectively, aim to lose no more than 1lb to 2lb a week. You may lose a little more than this when you first start dieting due to a loss of water as well as fat. But if you regularly lose more than 2lb a week, increase your calorie intake slightly - if you lose weight too quickly you're far more likely to put it back on again. A slow, steady loss is the answer - you'll be far more likely to keep the weight off once you've lost it.

BREAKFASTS
(200 calories)

Bacon butty
Grill 2 lean rashers back bacon and serve in 1 wholemeal bread roll with 1 grilled sliced tomato

Hot buttered crumpets
Top 2 toasted crumpets with 1½tsp butter

Porridge and honey
Heat 25g/1oz porridge oats with 150ml/¼pt skimmed milk for about five minutes. Stir in 1tsp runny honey and 1tbsp raisins

Croissant and hot chocolate
Warm 1 small croissant and serve with 2tsp no-added sugar jam and 1 sachet low-calorie instant hot chocolate

Fruit loaf
Serve 50g/2oz fruit loaf with 2tsp low-fat spread

Poached egg on toast
Poach 1 medium egg and serve on 1 medium slice wholemeal toast. Plus 115ml/4floz unsweetened orange juice

Wheat biscuits
Serve 2 wheat biscuits with 150ml/¼pt skimmed milk. Plus 1 satsuma

Yoghurt with banana
Slice 1 medium banana and serve with 150ml pot plain yoghurt

LIGHT MEALS
(300 calories)

Tasty toasties
2 medium slices wholemeal toast with 2tsp low-fat spread. Serve with one of these fillings and 'free' salad:
■ Cheese and onion: 40g/1½oz reduced-fat Cheddar cheese and 4 spring onions
■ Tuna mayo: mix together 65g/2½oz tuna canned in brine, diced cucumber, and 1tbsp each of reduced-calorie mayonnaise and low-fat plain yoghurt
■ Cheese and ham: 25g/1oz reduced-fat cheese with 40g/1½oz wafer thin ham
■ Soft cheese and smoked salmon: 50g/2oz low-fat soft cheese and 25g/1oz smoked salmon
■ Mackerel in tomato sauce: 50g/2oz mackerel canned in tomato sauce

Cheese omelette
Beat 2 medium eggs with 1tbsp water. Slice and poach 50g/2oz mushrooms. Heat 1tsp oil in a non-stick pan then pour in the eggs. Add mushrooms when almost set. Sprinkle over 25g/1oz grated reduced-fat Cheddar cheese. Serve with 'free' salad

Warming winter soup
500ml bottle of minestrone soup served with 1 wholemeal roll

Jacket potatoes
Bake a 200g/7oz potato, raw weight, top with one of the following, and serve with 'free' vegetables:
■ Baked beans: 200g can baked beans in tomato sauce

LIGHT MEALS (continued)

■ Cheese and tomato: 40g/1½oz grated reduced-fat cheese with 2 sliced tomatoes
■ Cottage cheese and pineapple: 150g/5oz cottage cheese mixed with 1 pineapple ring canned in fruit juice
■ Chicken and coleslaw: 115g/4oz reduced-calorie coleslaw and 50g/2oz chicken breast

Sardines on toast
Top 1 medium slice wholemeal toast with 1tsp low-fat spread and 125g can sardines in tomato sauce. Serve with 'free' salad

Hot beef baguette
Grill a 75g/3oz thin steak for a few minutes each side and serve in a 50g/2oz baguette with 'free' salad and 1tbsp creamed horseradish

Cauliflower cheese
Boil or steam 275g/10oz cauliflower. Place in an ovenproof dish and pour over 1 serving perfect reduced-fat cheese sauce (see recipe, below). Brown under the grill and serve with 25g/1oz crusty bread and 'free' vegetables

---

PERFECT REDUCED-FAT CHEESE SAUCE FOR ONE

■ 6.2g fat and 140 calories per portion

Melt 7g/¼oz low-fat spread in a non-stick pan and gradually add 7g/¼oz plain flour, stirring continuously. Slowly add 100ml/3½floz skimmed milk and then let the sauce simmer for 2 minutes. Add 15g/½oz grated reduced-fat Cheddar cheese, 1 bay leaf and freshly ground black pepper. Remove the bay leaf and serve.

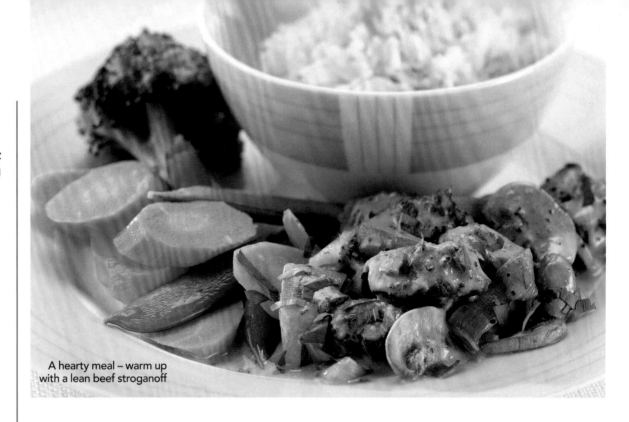

A hearty meal – warm up with a lean beef stroganoff

MAIN MEALS
(400 calories)

Bacon pasta
Grill and chop 2 rashers lean back bacon. Slice 2 open cap mushrooms. Poach and drain. Mix with 1 serving perfect reduced-fat cheese sauce (see recipe, left) and season with pepper. Boil 50g/2oz spaghetti, raw weight, and mix together. Serve with 'free' vegetables

Roast dinner and chocolate sponge
Serve 75g/3oz lean roast beef, pork, lamb or skinless chicken with 'free' vegetables, 115g/4oz boiled potatoes, raw weight, and 2tbsp fat-free gravy. Follow with 1 portion chocolate sponge pudding with strawberries with 2tbsp fat-free plain fromage frais

Cheesy mash and beans
Boil 275g/10oz potato, raw weight, and mash with 1 level tsp low-fat spread and 25g/1oz grated reduced-fat Cheddar cheese. Serve with 115g/4oz baked beans in tomato sauce and 'free' vegetables

Vegetable curry
■ Serves 4
Heat 1tsp oil in a pan, add 1 chopped medium onion, 1 clove crushed garlic and 1tsp hot curry powder. Fry until the onions are soft. Add 150g/5oz each of cauliflower, cubed raw potato, 25g/1oz split red lentils, and stir for a minute. Add a 400g can chopped tomatoes, 50g/2oz frozen peas and one cup of water. Bring to the boil, simmer for 20 minutes then add 2tbsp crème fraiche. Boil 115g/4oz rice, raw weight, then drain. Serve 1 portion of each. Follow with 1 small pot of diet yoghurt. You can freeze the rest of this dish for another time

Beef stroganoff
■ Serves 4
Heat 2tsp oil in a non-stick pan and gently fry 1 onion until brown. Cube then brown 450g/1lb lean rump steak. Add 115g/4oz mushrooms, sliced, 4tbsp beef stock, 2tbsp mustard and 2tsp coarse ground black peppercorns. Cook for 5 minutes, add 2tbsp brandy and stir in 75g/3oz reduced-fat crème fraiche. Simmer for 15 minutes. Meanwhile, boil 175g/6oz rice, raw weight, then drain. Serve 1 portion of each with 'free' vegetables. You can freeze the rest of the dish for another time

Sausage, beans and mash
Grill 2 low-fat pork sausages. Meanwhile, boil 200g/7oz potato, raw weight, and mash with 1tbsp skimmed milk. Sprinkle the mash with chopped fresh parsley and serve with the sausages and 50g/2oz baked beans in tomato sauce

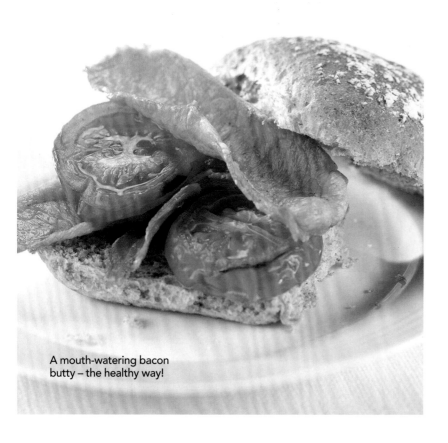

A mouth-watering bacon butty – the healthy way!

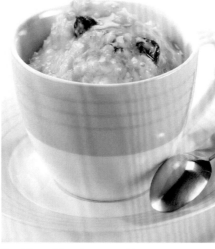

Porridge with sultanas and honey – a delicious breakfast

Cheese, ham and vegetable pizza
Top 2 mini cheese and tomato pizzas with sliced button mushrooms, ½ red pepper and 50g/2oz lean ham. Cook according to instructions. Serve with 'free' salad

Fish and chips
Bake 150g/5oz low-fat oven chips and grill 1 frozen breaded cod steak. Serve with 'free' vegetables

Salmon salad
Poach or grill a 75g/3oz salmon fillet and serve with 2tbsp reduced-calorie mayonnaise, 'free' salad and a 200g/7oz jacket potato, raw weight

Liver and onions and chocolate mousse
Heat 1tsp oil in a non-stick pan and gently fry 75g/3oz thinly-sliced lamb's liver and 1 small sliced onion for about 5 minutes. Bake/boil 200g/7oz potatoes, raw weight, and serve together with 'free' vegetables. Follow with 1 small pot low-fat chocolate mousse

SNACKS & PUDDINGS
(250 calories)

SWEET
Rice pudding and fruit
Serve 150g pot low-fat rice pudding with 1 apple, 1 pear and 1 satsuma

Chocolate sponge pudding with strawberries
Cook 1 individual low-fat chocolate sponge pudding according to manufacturer's instructions and serve with a few sliced strawberries

Biscuits and cakes
Choose ONE of the following:
3 plain digestive biscuits plus 1 satsuma
4 malted milk/round rich tea biscuits plus 1 orange
2 chocolate mini rolls
2 chocolate digestives plus
    1 small banana
    1 iced bun
    2 jam tarts
    50g/2oz angel cake

Banana custard
Serve a 150g pot low-fat custard with 1 large banana

Treacle sponge
Serve 100g/3½oz canned treacle sponge pudding with 2tbsp half cream

Bread and butter pudding
Serve a 150g/5oz portion bread and butter pudding with 1tbsp single cream

SAVOURY
Pasta bake
Combine 115g/4oz cooked pasta shapes and a selection of cooked vegetables in an ovenproof bowl. Pour over 1 serving perfect reduced-fat cheese sauce. Grill for a few minutes and serve

Jacket potato and ratatouille
Heat 200g can ratatouille Provençale and serve with 200g/7oz jacket potato, raw weight

Baked beans on toast
Top 1 medium slice wholemeal toast with 1 level tsp low-fat spread and 200g can baked beans in tomato sauce

Cheese and ham on toast
Toast 2 medium slices wholemeal bread and top them with 25g/1oz lean ham and 25g/1oz reduced-fat Cheddar cheese. Place under a hot grill for a few minutes. Serve with 'free' salad

Alcohol
Small glass of wine or lager, beer or cider, or 2 x 25ml measures spirit with diet mixers. Plus a small packet of crisps

Fruit
Serve as a fruit salad or eat separately:
1 small banana, 1 kiwi fruit, 1 orange, 1 apple and 1 pear

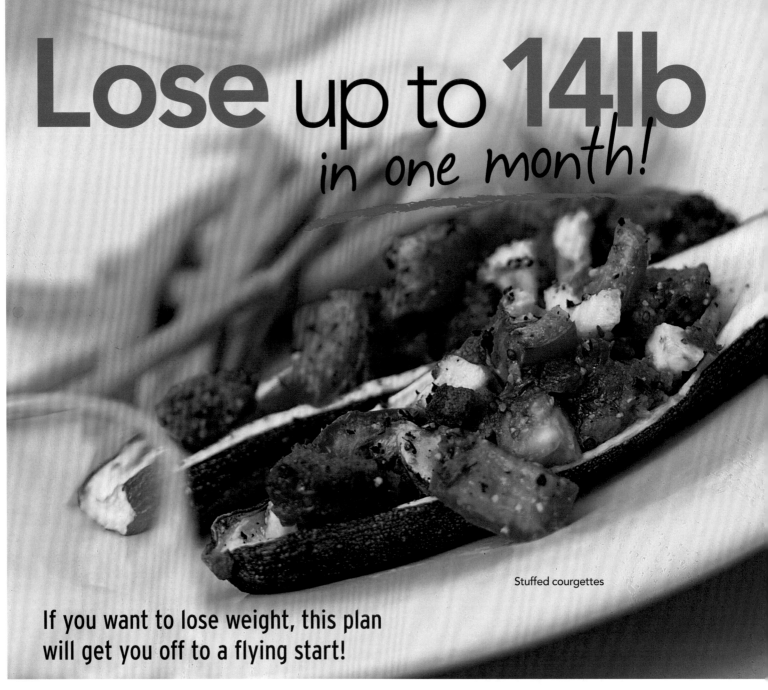

Lose up to 14lb
in one month!

Stuffed courgettes

If you want to lose weight, this plan will get you off to a flying start!

It's so simple...

Want to diet but can't muster up the energy to get started? We have the solution. All you need to do is arm yourself with our shopping list, buy what's on it, then follow the one-week menu through four cycles – and watch the weight fall off!

What do I do?

● Each day, have one breakfast, one light meal and one main meal, plus one, two or three snacks, depending on your allowance (see *How many calories do I need?*).

● On top of any milk used in the menus, have 275ml/½pt skimmed milk a day for tea and coffee, or two diet yoghurts, for

vital calcium.

● Drink unlimited amounts of water, coffee, tea (including herbal teas), Bovril and Marmite, low-cal or diet squashes and fizzy drinks.

● Eat all the meals and snacks listed for the week. Tick them off as you go so you don't repeat it.

● After one week, repeat the process for another three weeks.

How much will I lose?

In one week, you can expect to lose up to 3lb-4lb, so in a month you could lose up to 1st. In the long term, aim to lose 1lb-2lb a week. You may lose more at first, due to losing water as well as fat. If you regularly lose more than 2lb a week, you'll be losing muscle, which is not good for your health.

Be prepared

One of the best ways to stick to a diet is to plan your meals and snacks ahead of time and make a list. That way, when you're shopping, you're not tempted to buy 'off' the list. This simple plan takes care of all this for you by providing a weekly menu plan and a list of food you need to buy.

Copy *Your basic shopping list*, and take it to your local supermarket. For Plan A, simply buy everything on *Your basic shopping list*, and do not buy any *Extras*.

For Plan B, buy everything on *Your basic shopping list* plus the items on the *Extras* list. For Plan C, buy the *Extras* listed for Plan B and Plan C.

Off to the shops

Your basic shopping list, contains all the food you need for one week, except for a few store cupboard items. Most of the food can be bought in one trip but some may need to be picked up closer to the time of eating or stored in the freezer. Some of the food items, such as the frozen vegetables, are sold in bigger packs than you need for the week. Either use them in family meals or else they should last you the month.

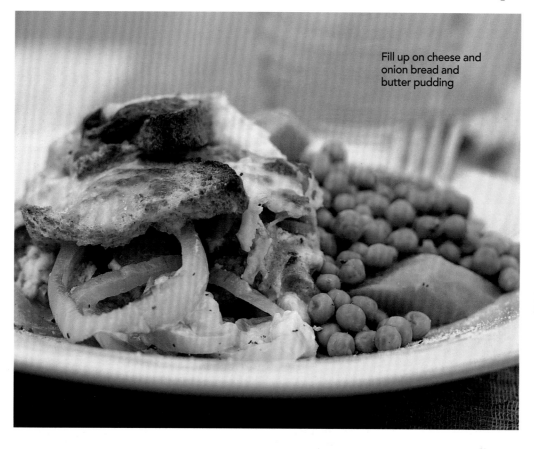

Fill up on cheese and onion bread and butter pudding

In the store cupboard Check you have these foods in stock

One-cal spray vegetable oil	Fat-free chicken gravy granules	Reduced-fat mayonnaise
Low-fat spread	Vegetable stock cubes	Fat-free vinaigrette
Jam	Wholegrain mustard	Black mustard seeds
Tomato purée	Dried thyme	Coffee, tea and diet drinks
Dried mixed herbs	Tomato ketchup	Paprika
English mustard	Cornflour	Vegetable or sunflower oil

How many calories do I need?

Your calorie allowance depends on how much weight you want to lose.
- **Less than 1st: Follow Plan A**
- **Between 1st and 3st: Follow Plan B**
- **More than 3st: Follow Plan C**

PLAN A: This is the basic diet and it provides an average of 1,250 calories per day. You need to buy everything on the shopping list, but not the *Extras*. Eat all the meals and snacks listed over a week.

PLAN B: On top of the basic diet, you need to eat one extra 250-calorie snack every day. Add *Extra shopping list Plan B*, to your basic list.

PLAN C: On top of the basic diet, you need to eat two extra 250-calorie snacks (500 cals) a day. So add *Extra shopping list Plan B and Plan C*, to your basic shopping list.

Your basic shopping list

Milk and dairy products
2.3ltr/4pt skimmed milk
125g pot diet yoghurt
150g/5oz low-fat natural yoghurt
75g/3oz half-fat mature Cheddar
115g/4oz low-fat soft cheese

Canned and dried foods
115g/4oz corned beef
300g can mixed beans
50g/2oz sweetcorn
150g/5oz tuna in brine, drained
1 x 400g and 1 x 200g can chopped tomatoes

Meat, fish and eggs
225g/8oz turkey mince
75g/3oz pack smoked mackerel fillets
4 rashers lean back bacon
150g/5oz cod fillet
50g/2oz ham
225g/8oz low-fat sausages
5 medium eggs

Cereal, bread, pasta, rice
750g box bran flakes,
Loaf wholemeal bread (medium slice)
3 wholemeal rolls
175g/6oz pasta shapes
100g/3½oz rice

Fruit and vegetables
5 apples
1 satsuma

2 small bananas
1 lemon
115g/4oz broccoli
3 x 200g/7oz baking potatoes
450g/1lb old potatoes for mashing
450g/1lb small new potatoes
4 onions
¼ savoy cabbage
½ leek
3 medium carrots
115g/4oz swede
115g/4oz parsnip
2 medium courgettes
25g/1oz button mushrooms
3 round lettuces for salads
1 red pepper
2 cucumbers
10 tomatoes
150g/5oz French beans
1 bulb of garlic
450g/1lb frozen mixed vegetables
450g/1lb frozen peas
150ml/¼pt unsweetened orange juice

Snacks
2 wholemeal fruit scones
3 wholemeal bread rolls
4 small bananas
2 apples
4 satsumas
75g/3oz canned tuna in brine
75g/3oz half-fat Cheddar cheese

Extras shopping list

Plan B
Add the following to your basic shopping list
2 x 200g MullerLight Mousses
2 McVitie Go Ahead Choc Chip Cake Bars
2 Options Pleasure chocolate drinks
4 mini pack Cadbury dairy fingers
1 apple, 2 oranges and 1 pear
2 Kit-Kats (4 finger)

Plan C
Add the following, plus the items for Plan B above, to the basic list
1 x 200g pot Muller Rice
50g/2oz dried apricots
2 x Frusli bars
2 regular packs Golden Lights
225g/8oz vanilla ice cream
2 small bananas, 1 apple and 2 satsumas

BREAKFASTS
Cereal and orange juice
4tbsp bran flakes with 150ml/¼pt skimmed milk, plus 150m/¼pt orange juice ☐

Bacon butty
Grill 2 rashers lean bacon and serve in a wholemeal roll with 1 tomato, sliced, unlimited lettuce and 1tbsp tomato ketchup ☐ ☐

Scrambled eggs on toast
Scramble 2 medium eggs with 1tsp low-fat spread and 1tbsp skimmed milk and serve with 1 medium slice wholemeal toast ☐ ☐

Cereal, banana and yoghurt
3tbsp bran flakes mixed with 1 small banana, sliced, and 5tbsp low-fat natural yoghurt ☐ ☐

LIGHT MEALS
Jacket potato with tuna
Bake a 200g/7oz potato. Top with 75/3oz tuna canned in brine, 1tbsp sweetcorn and 1tbsp reduced-fat mayonnaise ☐

Tuna and bean salad
Mix together 75g/3oz tuna canned in brine with ½ x 300g can mixed beans, drained, unlimited cucumber, diced, 1 tomato, chopped, and fat-free vinaigrette. Serve with 1 wholemeal roll ☐

Toasted cheese and ham sandwich
Toast 2 medium slices wholemeal bread. Fill with 25g/1oz each of ham and half-fat Cheddar cheese, grated. Serve with a salad of unlimited lettuce and cucumber, and 1 tomato, sliced ☐

Smoked mackerel salad
Serve 75g/3oz smoked mackerel with a salad of unlimited lettuce and cucumber, and 1 tomato, plus 1 slice bread ☐

Ham and mustard sandwich Spread 2 medium slices wholemeal bread with 1tsp low-fat spread and a scraping of English mustard. Fill with 25g/1oz ham. Serve with a salad of unlimited lettuce and cucumber, and 1 tomato ☐

Pasta and sweetcorn salad
Cook 50g/2oz pasta in lightly salted water, and drain. Mix together with 2tbsp sweetcorn and 1tbsp reduced-fat mayonnaise. Serve with a salad of unlimited lettuce and cucumber, and 1 tomato. Plus 1 satsuma ☐

Jacket potato and cheese
Bake a 200g/7oz potato. Top with 25g/1oz half-fat Cheddar, grated. Serve with a salad of unlimited lettuce and cucumber, and 1 tomato, sliced ☐

MAIN MEALS
Vegetable pasta
Boil 50g/2oz pasta and mix with half the tomato sauce (see *Recipes*) and 4tbsp frozen mixed veg, cooked. Serve with a salad of lettuce, cucumber and 1 tomato. Plus 1 pot diet yoghurt ☐

Turkey burgers with garlic mash
See *Recipes*. Plus 1 apple ☐

Pasta and tomato sauce
Boil 50g/2oz pasta. Top with 1 serving tomato sauce (see *Recipes*), sprinkled with 25g/1oz half-fat Cheddar, grated. Serve with 115g/4oz broccoli, steamed. Plus 1 apple ☐

Cheese and onion bread and butter pudding
See *Recipes*. Serve with 115g/4oz carrots and 4tbsp frozen peas, steamed. Plus 1 apple ☐

Sausage casserole
See *Recipes*. Serve with 115g/4oz carrots (raw weight), steamed. Plus 1 apple ☐

Stuffed courgette
See *Recipes*. Plus 1 satsuma ☐

Grilled cod and vegetables
Grill 150g/5oz skinless cod fillet, and serve with 4tbsp frozen mixed veg, cooked, and 200g/7oz boiled potatoes. Plus 1 apple ☐

SNACKS
Cheese roll
Fill 1 wholemeal roll with 1tsp low-fat spread and 40g/1½oz half-fat Cheddar ☐ ☐

Fruit selection
2 small bananas, 1 apple and 2 satsumas ☐ ☐

Tuna roll
Fill 1 wholemeal roll with 75g/3oz tuna in brine and 1½tbsp reduced-fat mayonnaise ☐

Scone with jam
1 wholemeal fruit scone with 2tsp low-fat spread and 4tsp jam ☐

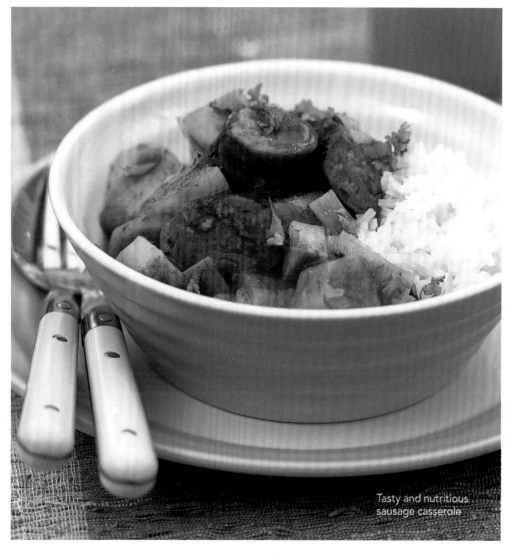
Tasty and nutritious sausage casserole

FOOD STYLING: SALLY MANSFIELD. PHOTOGRAPHY: JANINE HOSEGOOD

RECIPES: ALL MAKE 2 SERVINGS

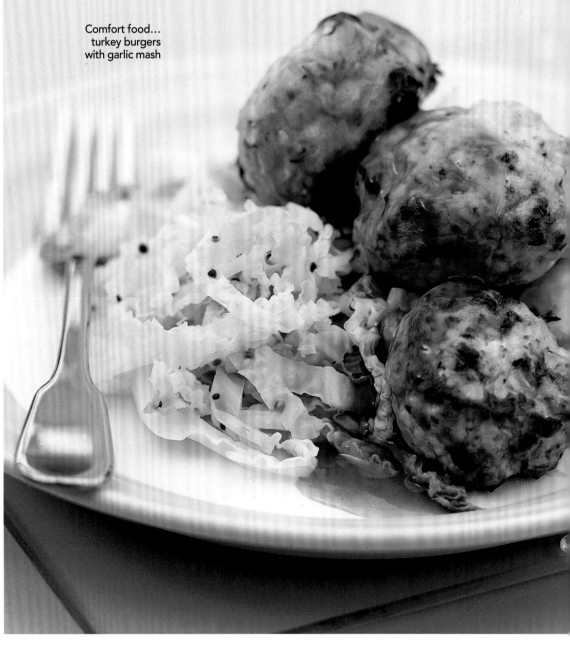

Comfort food...
turkey burgers
with garlic mash

Tomato sauce

Heat 1tsp oil in a nonstick pan and add 1
onion, sliced, 1 red pepper, diced, and 1
clove garlic, crushed. Stir and add a 400g
can chopped tomatoes, ½tsp dried mixed
herbs and 2tbsp tomato purée. Simmer for
20 minutes. Divide the mixture into two and
refrigerate or freeze.

Stuffed courgettes

- **Preparation: 20 minutes**
- **Cooking: 40 minutes**

■ 2 medium courgettes
■ Salt and pepper
■ Few sprays one-calorie oil

■ 115g/4oz lean corned beef
■ 25g/1oz button mushrooms, sliced
■ ½tsp wholegrain mustard
■ ¼tsp dried thyme
■ 1tsp tomato ketchup
■ 1 tomato, chopped
■ 450g/1lb small new potatoes
■ 150g/5oz French beans

1 Preheat the oven to 200°C/400°F/ gas
mark 6. Halve the courgettes lengthways
and scoop out the flesh. Chop half the flesh
and put in a bowl.

2 Place the skins on a nonstick baking sheet.
Season and spray with a little oil. Bake for
20 minutes.

3 Dice the corned beef and mix with the courgette flesh, mushrooms, mustard, thyme, ketchup and tomatoes. Take the skins from the oven and pile in filling. Season and bake for 20 minutes.

4 Boil the potatoes for 20 minutes and steam beans for 10 minutes. Drain and serve with the stuffed courgettes.

Turkey burgers with garlic mash

- **Preparation: 10 minutes**
- **Cooking: 22 minutes**

- ½ small onion, chopped
- 225g/8oz turkey mince
- ½ tsp lemon juice
- 1½tsp tomato purée
- 1tsp mixed dried herbs
- Salt and pepper
- Few sprays one-calorie oil
- 2 garlic cloves
- 450g/1lb potatoes, peeled
- 75ml/3floz skimmed milk
- 1½tbsp low-fat spread
- ¼ savoy cabbage
- ½tsp black mustard seeds
- 75ml/3floz fat-free chicken gravy to serve (optional)

1 Preheat the oven to 200°C/400°F/ gas mark 6. Put the onion, mince, lemon juice, purée and herbs in bowl. Season and mix to form a paste. Divide into 3 burgers. Spray a nonstick baking sheet with oil. Set the burgers on top.

2 Wrap the garlic in foil. Bake with the burgers for 15 minutes.

3 Chop the potatoes and boil for 20 minutes in lightly salted water. Drain and mash. Take the garlic from the oven, returning the burgers, and bake for a further 5 minutes. Squeeze the garlic into the mash with the milk and low-fat spread, and beat well. Keep hot.

4 Shred the cabbage, plunge into a pan of freshly boiled water and drain. Spray a nonstick frying pan or wok with oil and stir-fry the cabbage with the mustard seeds for 2 minutes.

5 Serve the burgers, mash and cabbage with the chicken gravy.

Cheese and onion bread and butter pudding

- **Preparation: 10 minutes, plus standing time**
- **Cooking: 40 minutes**

- Few sprays one-calorie spray oil
- 2 small onions
- 3 medium slices wholemeal bread
- 15g/½oz low-fat spread
- 115g/4oz low-fat soft cheese
- 50g/2oz reduced-fat mature Cheddar cheese, grated
- 1 medium egg
- 75ml/3floz skimmed milk
- 75ml/3floz water
- Salt and pepper
- Sprinkling of paprika
- 4tbsp frozen mixed vegetables

1 Preheat the oven to 180°C/350°F/ gas mark 4. Heat a nonstick frying pan and spray with a little oil. Slice the onion and cook, covered, until golden.

2 Lightly grease the base and sides of 275ml/½pt ovenproof dish. Spread the bread with the low-fat spread and cut each slice into four triangles. Arrange in the dish, spread side up, with the onions. Beat together the soft cheese, Cheddar, egg, milk and water. Season and pour over the bread. Leave to stand for 15 minutes.

3 Place the dish in a roasting tin half-filled with hot water. Bake for 40 minutes or until golden. Serve sprinkled with paprika and mixed vegetables.

Sausage casserole

- **Preparation: 15 minutes**
- **Cooking: 30 minutes**

- Few sprays one-calorie spray oil
- ½ medium leek
- 1 medium carrot
- 115g/4oz swede
- 115g/4oz parsnip
- 225g/8oz low-fat sausages
- ½ vegetable stock cube
- 15g/½oz casserole sauce mix
- 200g/7oz chopped tomatoes
- Salt and pepper
- 100g/3½oz rice (raw weight)

1 Spray a large nonstick saucepan with the oil. Chop the leek, carrot, swede and parsnip. Place in the pan and cook, covered, for 10 minutes.

2 Meanwhile, grill the sausages for 10 minutes. Halve the sausages and add to the vegetables with the stock cube, casserole sauce and tomatoes.

3 Add a little water to moisten. Season and cook, covered, for 20 minutes. Boil the rice in lightly salted water for 15 minutes.

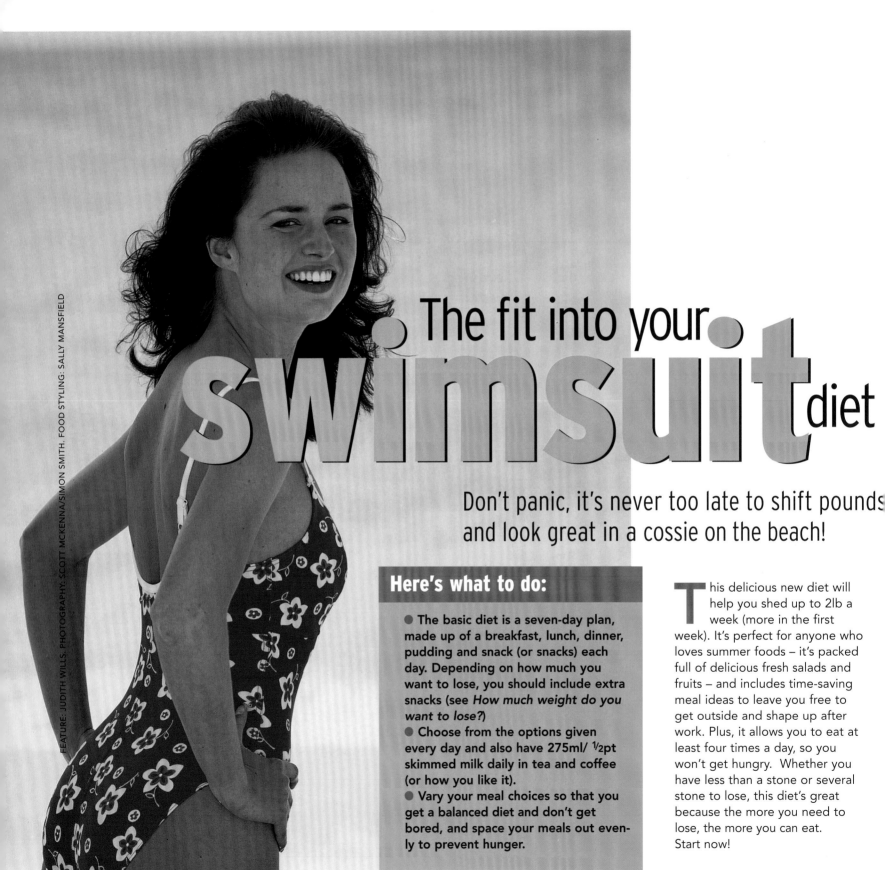

FEATURE: JUDITH WILLS. PHOTOGRAPHY: SCOTT MCKENNA/SIMON SMITH. FOOD STYLING: SALLY MANSFIELD

The fit into your swimsuit diet

Don't panic, it's never too late to shift pounds and look great in a cossie on the beach!

Here's what to do:

● The basic diet is a seven-day plan, made up of a breakfast, lunch, dinner, pudding and snack (or snacks) each day. Depending on how much you want to lose, you should include extra snacks (see *How much weight do you want to lose?*)

● Choose from the options given every day and also have 275ml/ ½pt skimmed milk daily in tea and coffee (or how you like it).

● Vary your meal choices so that you get a balanced diet and don't get bored, and space your meals out evenly to prevent hunger.

This delicious new diet will help you shed up to 2lb a week (more in the first week). It's perfect for anyone who loves summer foods – it's packed full of delicious fresh salads and fruits – and includes time-saving meal ideas to leave you free to get outside and shape up after work. Plus, it allows you to eat at least four times a day, so you won't get hungry. Whether you have less than a stone or several stone to lose, this diet's great because the more you need to lose, the more you can eat. Start now!

How much weight do you want to lose?

- **Less than 1st:** follow the basic diet choosing one snack a day from the 100-calorie snacks or two a day from the 50-calorie snacks.
- **1st to 3st:** follow the basic diet but choose snacks from the 50-, 100- or 200-calorie snacks list, adding up to a total of 350 calories.

Example: one 200-calorie snack, one 100-calorie snack and one 50-calorie snack.
- **3st or more:** follow the basic diet but choose snacks adding up to a total of 600 calories. For example: three 200-calorie snacks OR two 200-calorie snacks and two 100-calorie snacks.

- **For all calorie levels:** Vary your choice of snacks. If you have more than 1st to lose, choose only one snack from the *Sweet treats and alcohol* list a day. If you take all your snacks in the form of sweets or alcohol you won't have a balanced diet.

7 easy breakfasts

approx 250 calories

STRAWBERRY YOGHURT 200ml/7floz low-fat natural bio yoghurt topped with 150g/5oz strawberries, 1tsp caster sugar and 1tsp sunflower seeds.

MUESLI AND FRUIT 50g/2oz no-added-sugar muesli with 115ml/4floz skimmed milk (extra to allowance); 1 nectarine.

YOGHURT AND FRUIT 200g Müllerlight yoghurt, 1 banana and a handful of cherries.

CEREAL AND TOAST 25g/1oz Special K Red Berries with 115ml/4floz skimmed milk (extra to allowance); plus 1 medium slice wholemeal toast with 1tsp low-fat spread and 2tsp reduced-sugar jam.

CEREAL AND FRUIT 2 Weetabix with 115ml/4floz skimmed milk (extra to allowance) and 1tsp caster sugar; plus 1 peach.

BOILED EGG AND TOAST 1 medium boiled egg; 1 medium slice wholemeal toast with 1tsp low-fat spread; 150ml orange juice.

YOGHURT AND BANANA 100g pot Low-Fat Yoghurt; plus 1 banana.

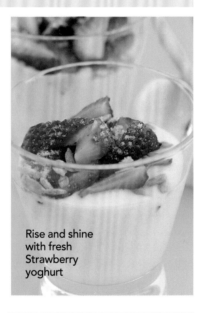

Rise and shine with fresh Strawberry yoghurt

Unlimited foods

To drink Tea or coffee with milk from your allowance, green or herbal tea or diet squash. Drink plenty of mineral water, too, especially on hot days or when exercising – aim for 2ltr a day.
To eat Liven up your meals by adding salad greens, fresh herbs and oil-free French dressing to whatever dishes you like.

7 quick lunches

PRAWN AND PASTA SALAD Toss 175g/6oz cooked pasta shapes with 75g/3oz peeled prawns, 6 halved cherry tomatoes, chopped cucumber and some fresh rocket or watercress leaves. Mix together 1tbsp reduced-calorie mayonnaise with 1tbsp low-fat bio yoghurt and a squeeze of lemon juice, and combine well with the salad.

approx 300 calories

FETA SALAD Slice 1 small gem lettuce and arrange on a serving plate with ½ red pepper, sliced, 1 tomato, chopped, a piece of cucumber, chopped, 1 spring onion, chopped and 2 stoned black olives, halved. Crumble over 40g/1½oz feta cheese and dress with oil-free French dressing. Serve with 1 small wholemeal roll spread with 1tsp low-fat spread. Plus 1 plum.

PARMA HAM SALAD Peel ¼ large ripe cantaloupe melon and cut it into cubes. Arrange on a serving plate with 50g/2oz Parma ham, torn roughly into strips. Serve with 1 small wholemeal roll spread with 1tsp low-fat spread.

HOUMOUS AND PITTA Take 1 wholemeal pitta, split in half and filled with 40g/1½oz reduced-fat, ready-made houmous and some chopped crisp salad items, such as cucumber, celery, carrot and lettuce heart. NOTE: You can thin the houmous a little with some oil-free French dressing if you prefer.

TURKEY BAGEL 1 bagel, split and spread with 2tsp reduced-calorie mayonnaise and filled with 25g/1oz wafer-thin turkey slices, 2tsp mango chutney and unlimited salad leaves. Plus a handful cherries or grapes.

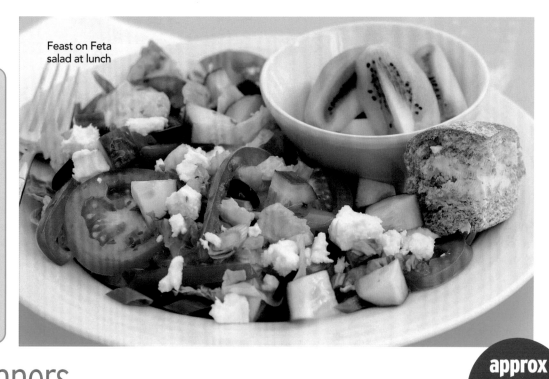
Feast on Feta salad at lunch

SANDWICH TO GO Any shop-bought or ready-made sandwich under 250 calories. Plus 1 apple, peach or nectarine.

HOT CIABATTA ROLL Halve a ciabatta roll and spread with 2tsp low-fat spread. Top with tomato, sliced, red onion, thinly sliced, and yellow pepper, thinly sliced, then finish with 65g/2½oz reduced-fat mozzarella cheese, sliced. Flash under the grill for a minute or two until the cheese has melted. Serve immediately. Follow with a 200g/7oz slice melon.

7 delicious dinners

approx 350 calories

PIZZA DELICATA
Spread 2tbsp low-fat soft cheese over a mini pizza base and top with ½ small ripe avocado, peeled and sliced. Top with tomato, thinly sliced, season with salt and pepper and bake at 200°C/400°F/gas mark 6 for 10 minutes or until the pizza is cooked and the top is bubbling. Serve immediately with green salad.

FRUITY CHICKEN COUSCOUS
Boil 65g/2½oz (dry weight) couscous for 10 minutes then fluff up. Meanwhile chop a cooked, skinned, 150g/5oz chicken breast fillet into small pieces and chop 3 ready-to-eat dried apricots, a piece of cucumber, and ½ yellow pepper. Stir everything into the couscous, together with a little oil-free French dressing.

CHEESY BAKED POTATO
1 x 250g baking potato, baked or microwaved. Split and fill with a mixture of 2tbsp low-fat soft cheese thoroughly combined with 1dsp salad cream, 50g/2oz cooked sweetcorn kernels and one spring onion, finely chopped. Serve with a salad made from a variety of green leaves, plus a sliced tomato.

LAMB AND MINT SAUCE
1 x 150g/5oz lamb steak, grilled or barbecued and served with 100g/3½oz new potatoes and a large portion of broccoli or spinach, plus 2tsp mint or redcurrant sauce.

SALMON PESTO
Take 1 x 125g/4½oz salmon steak, top with a mixture of 2tsp ready-made green pesto, 1 heaped tsp crushed pine nuts and a pinch of sea salt, and grill for 3-4 minutes on one side only until just cooked through and the topping browned. Serve

with a large mixed salad with oil-free dressing or with a selection of green vegetables.

MONKFISH KEBAB
Cut 200g/7oz monkfish (or other firm-fleshed white fish) into bite-sized cubes. Deseed a small red pepper and cut into bite-sized squares. Peel a small red onion and cut into thin bite-sized pieces. Thread the fish and vegetables onto one large or two small kebab sticks and brush with 1tsp olive oil. Grill or barbecue for 8 minutes, turning once, and serve with 1tbsp ready-made tomato salsa and 40g/1½oz (dry weight) pasta shapes, cooked.

QUICK SUPPER
Any ready meal of 325 calories per portion or less, served with broccoli, spring greens, mangetout, green beans or carrots, or with a mixed salad with oil-free French dressing.

Fast puddings

approx 150 calories

- Any medium pot Boots Shapers Dessert; 1 apple.
- 90g Cadbury's Light Trifle.
- 1/3 x sachet Angel Delight made with skimmed milk.
- 150g pot Ambrosia Low Fat Rice with 1tsp reduced-sugar jam.
- 60g pot Nestlé's Aero Mousse.
- 1 x 150g pot Onken Lite Mousse.

- 125g pot Rowntree's Jelly, plus 1 kiwi fruit.
- 100g/3½oz vanilla ice cream with 1dsp ready-made raspberry coulis.
- 150g/5oz fresh fruit salad topped with 1tbsp Greek yoghurt.
- 150g/5oz strawberries topped with 2 squirts half-fat aerosol cream.

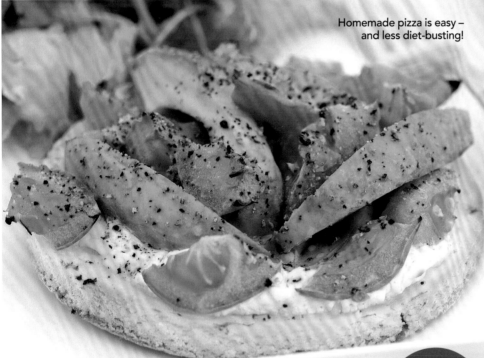

Homemade pizza is easy – and less diet-busting!

Sweet treats and alcohol

approx 200 calories

- 2 x 150ml glasses dry white wine.
- 1pt mild cider.
- 275ml bottle Bacardi Breezer.
- 2 pub measures of gin or vodka with tonic.
- 1 toasted teacake with 2tsp low-fat spread.

- 50g/2oz slice rich fruit cake.
- 2 Scotch pancakes spread with 1dsp fruit coulis.
- 1 Strawberry Cornetto ice cream.
- 1 x 175g pot Müller Fruit Corner yoghurt.

Snacks

EACH APPROXIMATELY 50 CALORIES
- 2 Rakusen's 99% Fat Free Crackers topped with 1tbsp low-fat soft cheese.
- 1 apple, peach, nectarine or small pear.
- 1 dark rye Ryvita topped with 2tsp runny honey.
- 1 x 125g pot Danone Activia 0% Fat Strawberry Yoghurt.
- 3 dried apricots.
- 1 slice Melba toast with 1tsp low-sugar jam.

EACH APPROXIMATELY 100 CALORIES
- 200g pot Müllerlight yoghurt.
- 1 Harvest bar.
- 1 medium slice bread with 1tsp low-fat spread and a little Marmite.
- 8 whole almonds.
- 2 reduced fat cheese triangles with 2 Rakusen's 99% Fat Free Crackers.
- 1 medium banana.

EACH APPROXIMATELY 200 CALORIES
- Sandwich made of 2 medium slices wholemeal bread with 1tsp low-fat spread, 2 reduced fat cheese triangles and 1tsp sweet pickle.
- 3 dark Ryvitas with 40g/1½oz half-fat Cheddar and 1 tomato.
- 1 medium bag crisps.
- 1 x 25g reduced-fat bag crisps and 1 large apple.
- 1 small wholemeal roll spread with 1tsp reduced-calorie mayonnaise and filled with 1 small hard-boiled sliced egg and cress or cucumber.
- 100g/3½oz cold cooked new potatoes, sprinkled with salt.
- 1 mini pitta with 2tbsp ready-made tzatziki or tomato salsa.
- 1 small bag Twiglets.
- 40g/1½oz no-added-sugar luxury muesli with 150ml/¼pt skimmed milk.

Eat more fat, lose weight

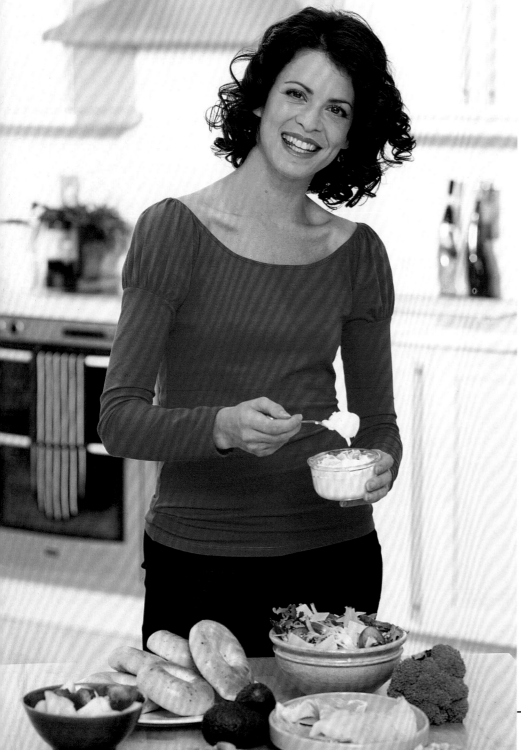

Struggling to stick to a regular low-fat diet? We've got the solution. New research shows that it's not only OK to include a bit more healthy fat in your diet, but that it helps you keep the weight off. We've created three simple diets based on this - work your way through them until you reach target

FEATURE: JENNETTE HIGGS. PHOTOGRAPHY: IAN HOOTON. STYLING: MARIA ZOKAS. HAIR & MAKE-UP: BRITTA D. RESEARCH PROVIDED BY THE AMERICAN PEANUT COUNCIL

Why this diet is different

It's unbelievable but true. New research shows that including more of the right kind of fat in your diet may actually help you lose weight – and keep it off in the long term. A recent study in the *International Journal of Obesity* involved 101 overweight men and women who followed either a very low-fat diet (20% calories from fat) or a moderate-fat diet (35% calories from fat) for 18 months. They all had the same amount of calories and had a low saturated fat intake, but those on the moderate-fat diet got their fats from healthier sources like peanuts, peanut butter and olive oil – the foods slimmers normally cut out.

While both groups dropped pounds, a year later the moderate-fat dieters had kept them off, but the low-fat dieters ended up 1lb heavier than when they'd started.

Isn't eating more fat bad for my health?

Government guidelines advise a total daily fat intake of 33% for a healthy heart. But it's now recognised that it's the type of fat you eat, not just the amount, that affects cholesterol levels and heart disease, says Dr Margaret Ashwell OBE, expert in nutrition and heart disease. 'Replacing saturated fat with unsaturated (as these diet plans do), is a more effective way of lowering the risk than just reducing the amount of fat in your diet.'

Doesn't this contradict Slimming's guidelines?

Slimming's philosophy is that, in order to lose weight, you need to burn more calories than you take in, and you should aim to get no more than 25% to 30% of these calories from fat. This new research is exciting as it shows you can follow a calorie-controlled diet with a slightly higher fat level (35% of calories from fat), and still slim.

'Because fat has more calories gram for gram than carbs or protein, it has been assumed that, for weight loss, fat levels should be kept low. But a slightly higher fat intake may help us stick to diets for longer. In the end, it's your total calorie intake, relative to your needs, that determines whether weight is lost or gained,' says Margaret.

With this in mind we've designed a three-step plan that will help you lose weight and keep it off. You should lose about ¹⁄₂lb to 1lb a week – and once you've started you won't want to stop.

> 'This research shows that people have to enjoy what they eat to stick with a diet. Diets that include moderate amounts of fat can be successful because they offer greater variety and taste good.'
>
> **Kathy McManus, the study's lead dietitian**

Healthy eating

Your 3-step plan

Step 1: Set your target weight

Refer to to the table below for your calorie allowance.

TARGET LOSS	CALORIE ALLOWANCE
Less than 1st	1,250 calories (see page 92)
1st to 3st	1,500 calories (see page 94)
More than 3st	1,800 calories (see page 96)

Step 2: Follow your plan to target

Every day we've listed the ingredients you need for your meals (all meals serve one). Eat/cook them how you like, but don't use any more oil than stated. At the end of the first week, repeat it or adapt it by swapping some choices as follows:

Breads, pasta, rice, potatoes: (wholegrain where possible): 2 small slices bread; 3 egg-sized potatoes; 150g/5oz cooked pasta; 100g/3¹⁄₂oz cooked rice; 4 crispbreads; 25g/1oz wholegrain cereals.

Main meal protein alternatives: 85g/3¹⁄₄oz lean meat or oily fish (uncooked weight); 100g/3¹⁄₂oz white fish (uncooked weight); 1 egg; 125g/4¹⁄₂oz cooked beans; 20g/³⁄₄oz cheese.

Fruit & vegetables: Fill up on any veg, salad or fruit (except potatoes). Fresh, frozen or canned. **Calcium:** 275ml/¹⁄₂pt skimmed milk or a low-fat yoghurt plus 150ml/¹⁄₄pt skimmed milk daily.

Healthy fats: include daily 3tsp olive, rapeseed or groundnut oil for salad dressings, stir-fries or marinades *and* 2tsp peanut butter, plus 25g/1oz nuts or peanuts. Here are some ideas:
● Use ground peanuts to thicken mild curries.
● Scatter salads and stir-fried vegetables with nuts.
● Garnish salads with toasted peanuts.

Step 3: Stay on target

When you've reached your goal, add 250 calories a day and weigh yourself after a week. If you're still losing weight, add another 250 calories a day the next week, and so on. When your weight levels out, that's how many calories you need to eat to stay slim. On average, this is around 1,940 calories for women.

250-calorie ideas include:
● **2 slices wholemeal toast** with 2tsp peanut butter
● **Wholemeal pitta bread** with 25g/1oz houmous and as much salad as you like
● **Sardine sandwich** made with 2 slices wholemeal bread and 50g/2oz sardines in tomato sauce
● **1 scrambled egg** made with 1tbsp skimmed
● **2 grilled fish fingers** in a wholemeal roll with 1tbsp ketchup
● **1 English muffin** with 2tsp low-fat spread and 2tsp reduced-sugar jam
● **50g/2oz chocolate bar**
● **1 fruit scone**

91

Less than 1st:
1,250 calories

This diet gives you around **34%** calories from fat each day

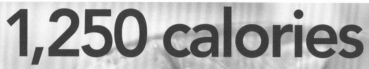

SEVEN-DAY MENU

MONDAY

Breakfast
- ½ cantaloupe melon
- 1 slice toast, 2tsp peanut butter
- 125g pot low-fat yoghurt

Lunch
Beef baguette: 75g/3oz baguette, 40g/1½oz cooked lean beef, sliced, 1 tomato, sliced, 25g/1oz watercress, 2 radishes, 1tsp mustard
- 1 satsuma

Snacks
- 25g/1oz roasted peanuts
- 125ml/4½floz skimmed milk (can be used in tea or coffee)

Dinner
Swordfish with vegetables and salad: 75g/3oz swordfish, 75g/3oz new potatoes, 25g/1oz mushrooms, 100g/3½oz asparagus, 75g/3oz salad greens, 1tbsp olive oil, 1tbsp vinegar
- 100g/3½oz strawberries

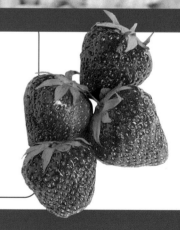

TUESDAY

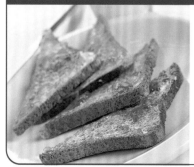

Breakfast
- 2 slices wholemeal toast, 2tsp peanut butter, 1tsp jam or honey
- 1 medium banana

Lunch
Chicken salad: 50g/2oz chicken breast, skinned, 65g/2½oz fresh spinach, 3 cherry tomatoes, halved, 1tsp olive oil, 1tbsp vinegar, ¼tsp sesame seeds, 2 medium breadsticks
- 3 fresh apricots

Snacks
- 25g/1oz roasted almonds
- 250ml/9floz skimmed milk

Dinner
Seafood stir-fry:
75g/3oz shrimps, 100g/3½oz broccoli, 40g/1½oz courgette, 25g/1oz red pepper, 2tsp groundnut oil, 100g/3½oz rice (dry weight), boiled
- 125ml/4½floz tomato juice

WEDNESDAY

Breakfast
- 25g/1oz bran cereal, 125ml/4^1/2floz skimmed milk, 100g/3^1/2oz raspberries
  - ^{1}/2 medium muffin, 1tsp peanut butter

Lunch
Turkey pocket: 1 wholemeal pitta bread, 50g/2oz turkey breast, sliced, 3 slices fresh tomato, 4 slices cucumber, 25g/1oz alfalfa sprouts or beansprouts, 2tsp mustard

Snacks
- 25g/1oz roasted macadamia nuts (seeds of the macadamia tree; available in supermarkets)
- 125ml/4^1/2floz skimmed milk

Dinner
Italian special: 115g/4oz wholemeal pasta, dry weight, 125g/4^1/2oz tomato-based pasta sauce, 75g/3oz green beans, 2tbsp Parmesan cheese, grated
- 40g/1^1/2oz salad, 2tsp olive oil, 1tbsp vinegar

New research shows that it's not only OK to include a little more healthy fat in your diet, but that it actually helps you keep the weight off

THURSDAY

Breakfast
- 1 medium wholewheat bagel, 1tbsp peanut butter
- 125ml/4^1/2floz orange juice

Lunch
Bean feast: 1 slice wholemeal bread, 100g/3^1/2oz baked beans in tomato sauce

- 50g/2oz green salad, 25g/1oz avocado, 1tsp olive oil, 1tbsp vinegar

Snacks
- 25g/1oz roasted mixed nuts
- 275ml/^{1}/2pt skimmed milk

Dinner
Chicken plate: 75g/3oz skinless chicken breast, 100g/3^1/2oz potato, baked in skin, 60g/2^1/4oz French beans, 75g/3oz broccoli, 25g/1oz mangetout, 1tsp olive oil
- ^{1}/2 pink grapefruit

FRIDAY

Breakfast
- 1 slice granary bread, 2tsp peanut butter, 150g/5oz blackberries, stewed with 1tsp sugar, 2tsp maple syrup

Lunch
Ham sandwich: 2 thin slices wholemeal bread, 50g/2oz extra-lean ham, 2tsp mustard, 2 lettuce leaves, 1 small tomato, sliced
- 1 kiwi fruit

Snacks
- 25g/1oz walnuts
- 150ml/^{1}/4pt skimmed milk

Dinner
Haddock with garlic spinach: 115g/4oz haddock, steamed, 25g/1oz basmati rice, boiled, 150g/5oz sweetcorn, boiled if fresh, 1 tomato, grilled, 1 clove garlic, fried in 1tbsp olive oil, 150g/5oz spinach, cooked (covered) for about 5 minutes and tossed in oil

SATURDAY

Breakfast
- 1 cereal wheat biscuit (such as Weetabix), with milk from daily allowance, ^{1}/2tbsp raisins, 1 sliced peach
- 1 medium slice wholemeal toast, 2tsp peanut butter

Lunch
Open sardine salad sandwich:

50g/2oz sardines, fresh, grilled or canned, 2 medium slices wholemeal bread, 1 small tomato, sliced, 4 lettuce leaves
- 1 medium orange

Snacks
- 25g/1oz roasted hazelnuts
- 150ml/^{1}/4pt skimmed milk

Dinner
Oven-roast pork and veg with fresh green salad: 75g/3oz pork tenderloin, sliced and roasted in a hot oven for 20 minutes, with 50g/2oz pasta, boiled, 50g/2oz courgettes, sliced, 50g/2oz beetroot, sliced, 60g/2^1/4oz mixed salad greens dressed with 2tsp olive oil and 1tbsp cider vinegar

SUNDAY

Breakfast
- 20g/^{3}/4oz bran cereal with milk from daily allowance
- 1 crumpet, toasted, 1tsp yeast extract (eg Marmite), 1tsp peanut butter
- 100g/3^1/2oz fresh fruit salad

Lunch
Muffin mix: 1 toasted medium wholemeal English muffin, 25g/1oz houmous, 2tsp peanut butter, 65g/2^1/2oz low-fat three bean salad, 150g/5oz tomatoes
- 1 low-fat yoghurt

Snack
- 40g/1^1/2oz peanut and raisin mix
- 250ml/9floz skimmed milk

Dinner
Chinese beef stir-fry: 75g/3oz trimmed lean beef, 60g/2^1/4oz broccoli, 50g/2oz carrots, 50g/2oz red pepper, all sliced and stir-fried in 2tsp groundnut oil, served with 20g/^{3}/4oz Chinese noodles (dry weight), cooked

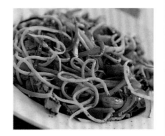

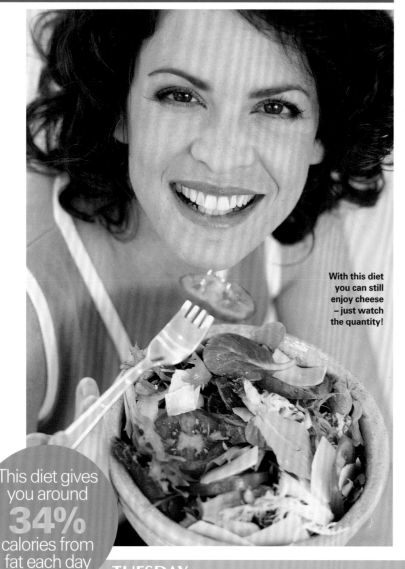

With this diet you can still enjoy cheese – just watch the quantity!

This diet gives you around **34%** calories from fat each day

1st to 3st:
1,500 calories

SEVEN-DAY MENU

MONDAY

Breakfast
- 1/2 cantaloupe melon
- 1 slice wholemeal toast, 2tsp peanut butter
- 125g pot low-fat yoghurt

Lunch
Soup and sarnie: 2 slices wholemeal bread, 25g/1oz reduced-fat Edam cheese, 1 small tomato, sliced, 1tsp mustard
- 225ml/8floz minestrone soup

Afternoon snacks
- 2 wholegrain crackers, 2tsp peanut butter
- 125ml/4½floz skimmed milk (can be used with tea and coffee)

Dinner
Fish with steamed veg: 115g/4oz swordfish, grilled or baked,150g/5oz new potatoes, with skins, 25g/1oz mushrooms, 75g/3oz asparagus, 75g/3oz mixed salad dressed with 1tbsp olive oil and 1tbsp vinegar
- 100g/3½oz strawberries

Evening snack
- 25g/1oz roasted peanuts

TUESDAY

Breakfast
- 2 large slices wholemeal toast, 3tsp peanut butter
- 1 medium banana

Lunch
Chicken and spinach salad: 50g/2oz cooked chicken breast, skinned, 50g/2oz fresh spinach leaves, drizzled with 2tsp olive oil and 1tbsp vinegar
- 1 sesame breadstick
- 1 medium orange

Afternoon snacks
- 25g/1oz roasted almonds
- 125ml/4½floz skimmed milk

Dinner
Shrimp stir-fry: 75g/3oz large shrimps, thawed, 75g/3oz broccoli, 25g/1oz red pepper, ¼ onion, 40g/1½oz courgette, all chopped and stir-fried in 1tbsp groundnut oil, served on 65g/2½oz brown rice (dry weight), boiled

Evening snack
- 125g pot fresh or frozen low-fat vanilla yoghurt

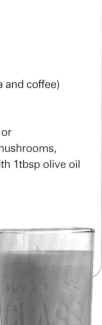

WEDNESDAY

Breakfast
- 25g/1oz bran cereal, 175ml/6floz skimmed milk, 100g/3½oz raspberries
- 1 wholemeal English muffin, 3tsp peanut butter

Lunch
Turkey salad pitta pocket: 1 wholemeal pitta, 50g/2oz turkey breast, sliced, 25g/1oz alfalfa or beansprouts, 3 slices tomato, 2tsp mustard
- 3 fresh apricots

Afternoon snacks
- 1 peach
- 125ml/4½floz skimmed milk (can be used in tea)

Dinner
Crab pasta: 50g/2oz pasta (dry weight), boiled, 75g/3oz crab meat, 75g/3oz green beans, sliced, 125g/4½oz tomato-based pasta sauce, 1tbsp Parmesan cheese, grated
- 40g/1½oz salad dressed with 1tbsp olive oil and 1tbsp vinegar

Evening snack
- 25g/1oz roasted macadamia nuts

THURSDAY

Breakfast
- 1 wholemeal bagel, 1tbsp peanut butter
- 1 banana, sliced
- 125ml/4½floz fresh orange juice

Lunch
Waldorf salad: 60g/2¼oz salad greens, 50g/2oz green apple, chopped, 25g/1oz mangetout, 20g/¾oz walnuts, 1tbsp olive oil, 1tbsp vinegar
- 1 slice wholemeal bread

Afternoon snacks
- 25g/1oz roasted mixed nuts
- 125ml/4½floz skimmed milk

Dinner
Grilled chicken and veg: 75g/3oz chicken breast, skinned, 185g/6½oz potato, baked, 75g/3oz broccoli,

Evening snacks
- 125g pot low-fat yoghurt
- 25g/1oz dates

FRIDAY

Breakfast
- 1 slice granary bread, 1tbsp peanut butter, 1tsp maple syrup, 185g/6½oz blackberries, stewed with 1tsp sugar

Lunch
Cheese and ham sarnie: 2 slices wholemeal bread, 50g/2oz lean ham, 25g/1oz Emmenthal cheese, sliced, 2 leaves lettuce, 1 small tomato, sliced, 2tsp mustard
- 1 kiwi fruit

Afternoon snacks
- 200g/7oz mandarin oranges in juice, 25g/1oz raisins
- 125ml/4½floz skimmed milk

Dinner
Fish and salad: 115g/4oz haddock, steamed, 20g/¾oz brown rice (dry weight), boiled, 150g/5oz sweetcorn, 150g/5oz sugar snap peas, 100g/3½oz spinach, 1 tbsp olive oil and 2tbsp vinegar

Evening snack
- 25g/1oz walnuts

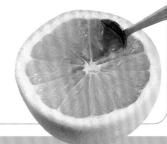

SATURDAY

Breakfast
- 200g/7oz porridge, made with water, 200ml/7floz skimmed milk, 2tbsp raisins
- 1 medium slice wholemeal toast, 2tsp peanut butter

Lunch
Sardine sarnie: 2 medium slices wholemeal bread, 50g/2oz sardines in oil, drained, 1 small tomato, 2tsp mustard

Afternoon snacks
- 1 grapefruit
- 250ml/9floz skimmed milk

Dinner
Pork special: 75g/3oz pork tenderloin, 50g/2oz brown rice (dry weight), boiled, 50g/2oz beetroot, 50g/2oz courgette, 60g/2¼oz mixed salad greens dressed with 1tbsp olive oil and 1tbsp cider vinegar

Evening snack
- 25g/1oz roasted hazelnuts

SUNDAY

Breakfast
- 1 egg, poached
- 2 slices wholemeal bread, 2tsp peanut butter

Lunch
Houmous roll and bean salad: 1 wholemeal roll, 50g/2oz houmous, 150g/5oz tomatoes, sliced, 60g/2¼oz low-fat three bean salad

Afternoon snacks
- 125g low-fat plain yoghurt, 1tsp honey
- 1 pear
- 125ml/4½floz skimmed milk

Dinner
Grilled salmon with couscous: 100g/3½oz salmon, grilled, 40g/1½oz couscous, dry weight, hydrated, 60g/2¼oz broccoli, 50g/2oz carrots, 60g/2¼oz cucumber, chopped, 20g/¾oz lettuce dressed with 2tsp olive oil and 1tbsp vinegar

Evening snack
- 40g/1½oz mixed peanuts and raisins

More than 3st:
1,800 calories

This diet gives you around **34%** calories from fat each day

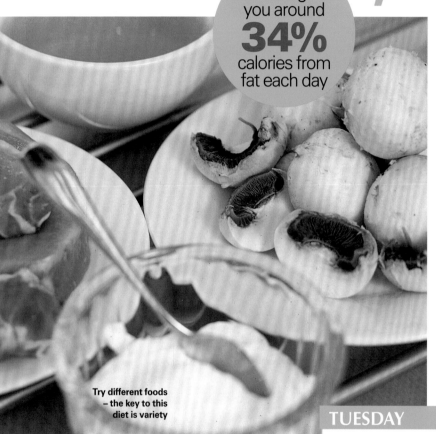

Try different foods – the key to this diet is variety

This new research is exciting as it shows you can follow a calorie-controlled diet with a slightly higher fat level (up to 35% of calories from fat) and still slim

SEVEN-DAY MENU

MONDAY

Breakfast
- 20g/³/₄oz porridge oats, cooked with water, 2tbsp raisins, 3 walnuts, halved, 125g/4¹/₂oz blackberries

Lunch
Salmon sandwich: 2 slices wholemeal bread, 50g/2oz canned salmon, 75g raw carrot, grated, 1tbsp reduced-calorie mayonnaise
- 1 medium peach

Afternoon snacks
- 25g/1oz mixed nuts
- 50g/2oz grapes

- 150ml/¹/₄pt skimmed milk (can be used with tea/coffee)

Dinner
Pork stir-fry: Stir-fry 85g/3¹/₄oz trimmed lean pork, sliced, 75g/3oz cauliflower, 75g/3oz courgette, in 2tsp olive oil. Serve with 35g/1¹/₄oz couscous (dry weight), hydrated, 50g/2oz salad greens, 3 tomato wedges, 15g/¹/₂oz avocado, 2tsp olive oil, 1tbsp vinegar

Evening snacks
- 1 small wholemeal roll
- 125g/4¹/₂oz raspberry sorbet

TUESDAY

Breakfast
- 1 medium slice wholemeal bread, 1tbsp peanut butter
- 175ml/6floz apple juice

Lunch
Beef salad sandwich: 2 medium slices wholemeal bread,

50g/2oz lean roast beef, 3 slices tomato, 2 lettuce leaves, 2tbsp reduced-calorie mayonnaise
- 1 medium orange

Afternoon snacks
- 25g/1oz walnuts
- 1 medium apple
- 150ml/¹/₄pt skimmed milk

Dinner
Baked fish: 100g/3¹/₂oz

haddock, baked, served with 65g/2¹/₂oz brown rice (dry weight), boiled, 90g/3¹/₄oz mixed veg, steamed or boiled, 40g/1¹/₂oz spinach leaves, 25g/1oz cucumber, sliced, 25g/1oz avocado, cubed, 4tsp olive oil, 1tbsp vinegar
- 125g citrus sorbet

Evening snack
- 125g pot low-fat yoghurt

WEDNESDAY

Breakfast
- 50g/2oz bran flakes, 125ml/4¹/₂floz skimmed milk, 50g/2oz strawberries
- 1 thick slice wholemeal toast, 1tsp jam

Lunch
Ham and cheese sandwich: 2 thick slices wholemeal bread, 65g/2¹/₂oz extra-lean ham, 20g/³/₄oz reduced-fat cheese, 4 slices beetroot, 2tsp reduced-calorie mayonnaise
- 200ml/7floz grapefruit juice

Afternoon snacks
- 25g/oz peanuts
- 125ml/4¹/₂floz skimmed milk

Dinner
Swordfish with courgettes and roasted pepper: 100g/3¹/₂oz swordfish, 160g/5³/₄oz new potatoes with skins, 60g/2¹/₄oz courgettes, 25g/1oz red pepper roasted with 1tbsp olive oil, 60g/2¹/₄oz salad greens in 1tbsp olive oil
- 2 plums

Evening snack
- 60g/2¹/₄oz wholemeal crackers

THURSDAY

Breakfast
- 40g/1¹/₂oz Raisin Wheats, 125ml/4¹/₂floz skimmed milk, 1 small banana
- 1 slice wholemeal bread, 3tsp honey

Lunch
Tuna pitta: 1 pitta, 50g/2oz tuna, 2 lettuce leaves, 3 slices tomato, 4 slices cucumber, 1tbsp mayonnaise
- 1 medium nectarine

Afternoon snacks
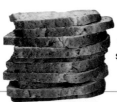
- 20g/³/₄oz almonds
- 125ml/4¹/₂floz skimmed milk

Dinner
Lamb stir-fry with spaghetti: 75g/3oz trimmed, lean lamb steak, 75g/3oz onion, 175g/6oz broccoli, 40g/1¹/₂oz mushrooms, 75g/3oz carrots, 75g/3oz spaghetti (dry weight), boiled, 75g/3oz salad greens, 40g/1¹/₂oz radishes, 2tbsp olive oil, 1tbsp vinegar

Evening snack
- 25g/1oz peanuts

FRIDAY

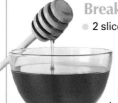

Breakfast
- 2 slices wholemeal bread, 1tbsp peanut butter, 2tbsp honey
- 200ml/7floz orange juice

Lunch
Mini-pizza: 1 wholemeal English muffin or roll, 25g/1oz reduced-fat cheddar, 1¹/₂tbsp tomato purée, 6 strips green pepper, 100g/3¹/₂oz canned baked beans, 2 slices fresh pineapple

Afternoon snack
- 25g/1oz pistachio nuts
- 125ml/4¹/₂floz skimmed milk

Dinner
Beef and bean stir-fry: 185g/6¹/₂oz potato, baked with 75g/3oz trimmed lean beef, 25g/1oz onion, 65g/2¹/₂oz green beans, all sliced and stir-fried in 2tsp olive oil, with 75g/3oz salad greens in 1tbsp olive oil and 1tbsp vinegar
- 170g/5³/₄oz apple, baked and sweetened with 2tsp sugar

Evening snack
- 1 wholemeal roll

SATURDAY

Breakfast
- 200g/7oz porridge made with 200ml/7floz skimmed milk, 20g/³/₄oz golden syrup, 10 raspberries

Lunch
Turkey salad: 90g/3¹/₄oz turkey breast, grilled, 25g/1oz salad greens, 25g/1oz ripe olives, 3 slices tomato, 2tsp olive oil, 1tbsp vinegar, 5 crackers

Afternoon snacks
- 1 large slice wholewheat bread, 2tsp Sun-Pat or Skippy peanut butter, 1tbsp jam
- 150ml/¹/₄pt skimmed milk

Dinner
Pasta with salad: 100g/3¹/₂oz-pasta (dry weight), 125ml/4¹/₂floz tomato-based pasta sauce, 20g/³/₄oz lean back bacon, chopped, 75g/3oz lettuce, 6 slices cucumber, 1tbsp olive oil
- 1 medium pear

Evening snack
- 25g/1oz peanuts

SUNDAY

Breakfast
- 2 slices wholemeal bread, 2tsp peanut butter, 1 banana, 8 strawberries, 1tsp honey

Lunch
Grilled chicken: 60g/2¹/₄oz chicken breast, grilled, 1¹/₂tbsp olive oil, 60g/2¹/₄oz spinach, 6 croutons, 1tbsp vinegar, 2 sesame breadsticks
- 125ml/4¹/₂floz apple juice

Afternoon snacks
- 25g/1oz peanuts
- 150ml/¹/₄pt skimmed milk

Dinner
Stir-fry with scallops: 1¹/₂tbsp olive oil, 25g/1oz onions, 60g/2¹/₄oz carrots, 25g/1oz yellow pepper, 60g/2¹/₄oz broccoli, all sliced and stir-fried with 75g/3oz scallops. Serve with 65g/2¹/₂oz long grain rice (dry weight), boiled

Evening snack
- 250g pot fat-free frozen yoghurt (any flavour)

You know that time of year. Summer holidays are a distant memory and suddenly Christmas is just around the corner. But don't panic if you think your favourite party outfit might be on the tight side. Start your diet now and go on to enjoy those parties, confident that you're looking good and feeling great

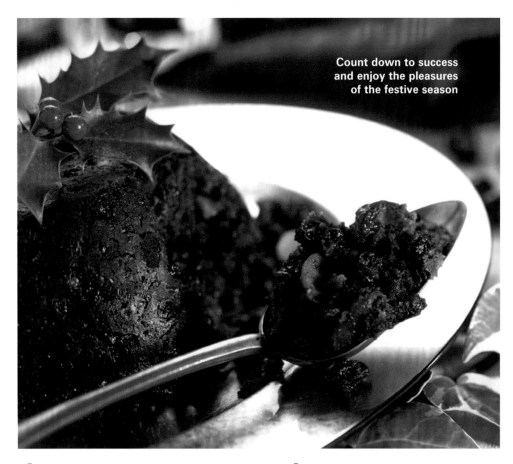

Count down to success and enjoy the pleasures of the festive season

21 day countdown
to Christmas

What do I do?

Follow the plan for 21 days

How much will I lose?

Up to 10lb

What's my calorie allowance?

Less than 1st to lose: 1,250
Between 1st and 3st to lose: 1,500
More than 3st to lose: 1,800

The plan – under 1st to lose

Every day have one breakfast, one light meal and one main meal, plus one or two snacks. You can eat your light meal at midday or in the evening – whichever suits you best. If you exercise regularly – which will help the weight loss and firm up your body – eat your snacks straight after you finish your exercise session.

The plan – more than 1st to lose

The same as if you've got under 1st to lose, plus up to 250 or 550 calories extra a day, depending on whether you need to lose 1st-3st or over 3st. This is best achieved by increasing your portions of carbohydrate-rich foods Here are some examples:

75g/3oz cooked pasta or rice	100 cals
125g/5oz cooked potato	100 cals
50g/2oz wholemeal roll or bap	125 cals
1 large wholemeal pitta bread	175 cals
1 slice wholemeal bread (medium slice, large loaf)	75 cals
30g serving bran flakes	100 cals
1 crispbread	30 cals

5 STEPS TO SUCCESS

1 Get your calcium
On top of any milk used in meals, every day have 275ml/½pt skimmed milk for tea and coffee or to drink on its own; or have two small pots of diet yoghurt or 150ml/¼pt skimmed milk and one small pot of diet yoghurt. These are all good sources of calcium, vital for strong bones and fat burning.

2 Drink plenty of fluids
Drink as much as you like of water, tea, coffee, herbal teas, Bovril or Marmite.

3 Eat up your veggies
You can have unlimited amounts of vegetables – raw or lightly cooked (boiled, steamed or microwaved) at all light and main meals. Vary the vegetables you eat on a daily basis, choosing from: **artichokes,** asparagus, **aubergines,** bean sprouts, **broccoli,** Brussels sprouts, **cabbage,** carrots, **cauliflower,** celery, **chicory,** courgettes, **cucumber,** fennel, **garlic,** gherkins, **green beans,** leeks, **lettuce,** mangetout, **marrow,** mushrooms, **onions,** peppers, **pumpkins,** radish, **spinach,** spring greens, **swede,** tomatoes, **turnip** and watercress.

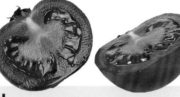

4 Make up a fruit bowl
Where the meal plans suggests a portion of fruit, choose one of the following: 1 medium apple ● 3 fresh apricots ● 1 bowl of berries (any variety or a mixture) ● 20-25 cherries ● 2 clementines, tangerines or satsumas ● 1 bowl of fresh fruit salad ● ½ grapefruit ● 15 grapes ● 2 kiwi fruits ● 1 large slice of melon ● 1 medium nectarine or peach ● 1 medium orange ● 1 medium pear ● 2 rings of pineapple ● 3 medium plums. Ideally choose fresh fruit but you can include the equivalent amount of canned fruit in natural juice – no syrup!

5 Love spices
Use as much as you like from the following list: **freshly ground black pepper,** garlic, **light soy sauce,** Worcestershire sauce, **Oriental fish sauce,** lemon juice and any fresh or dried herbs and spices. Try not to use salt in cooking or sprinkle it on food – let the herbs and spices give the flavours. Serve salads with a lemon juice and herb dressing or a tablespoon of fat-free vinaigrette dressing.

BREAKFASTS (300 CALS)

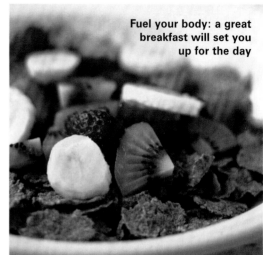
Fuel your body: a great breakfast will set you up for the day

TOAST AND JUICE (V)
Toast 2 medium slices from a large wholemeal loaf, spread one slice with 1tsp peanut butter and one with 1tsp of jam or honey. Plus 115ml/4floz unsweetened orange or grapefruit juice.

CEREAL AND FRUIT
Serve 40g/1½oz bran flakes or cornflakes with 150ml/¼pt skimmed milk. Plus 1 small, sliced banana and 115ml/4floz glass unsweetened orange or grapefruit juice.

ORANGE AND BANANA SMOOTHIE (V)
Place 1 chopped large ripe banana in a liquidiser or food processor. Juice 2 oranges (or alternately use 200ml/7floz unsweetened orange juice). Add a little orange juice to the banana and blend until smooth. Gradually add the remaining orange juice, 1tbsp lime juice, and 75ml/3floz low-fat natural yoghurt and continue to mix. Pour into a glass and drink at once!

BLT MUFFIN
Grill 2 slices back bacon, trimmed of fat, until crisp. Split and toast 1 English muffin, spread with 1tbsp light mayonnaise and arrange the bacon, some lettuce and 1 tomato sliced over the muffin halves. Serve with 115ml/4floz unsweetened orange or grapefruit juice.

CHEESY BAGEL (V)
Split 1 bagel and spread with 1tbsp low-fat soft cheese. Serve with 115ml/4floz unsweetened orange or grapefruit juice.

FRUITY PORRIDGE (V)
Add 25g/1oz porridge oats with 200ml/7floz skimmed milk to a pan and cook for 3-4 minutes, stirring continuously. When cooked, add 15g/½oz raisins and 1 small banana, chopped, and stir. Place in a bowl and add 1tbsp low-fat natural yoghurt. Serve with 115ml/4floz unsweetened orange or grapefruit juice.

MUESLI AND YOGHURT (V)
Serve 40g/1½oz muesli with 150ml/¼pt skimmed milk and 115ml/4floz unsweetened orange or grapefruit juice. Plus 1 115g/4oz pot low-fat fruit yoghurt.

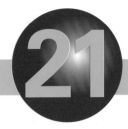

21 DAY COUNTDOWN

Where a quantity of food is given, measure it out using your kitchen scales or measuring jug – at least in the first week. Often people become overweight, not because they eat the wrong foods but because they just eat too much of the right foods.

If you find you're getting stuck on the diet, go back to weighing food again. Portions may have crept up in size without you realising.

Make a shopping list of the food you need for your diet and keep to it. Don't be tempted to buy things that aren't on the list – you'll only eat them!

Never go food shopping when you're hungry – the non-diet foods will seem even more appealing and you'll be more tempted to buy them.

Try not to eat on the move. Make a rule that from now on you will only eat sitting at a table. If you do just grab lunch on the run, it's less satisfying and although you may have consumed as many calories, you won't feel like you've had a proper meal.

Don't combine eating with other activities such as walking in the street, watching a film at the cinema or watching TV. Such mindless snacking can add up to lots of fat and calories each day, which you probably won't even remember eating.

Appreciate when you are starting to feel satisfied. That way you won't overeat. Remember, it takes 20 minutes for food to reach your stomach!

Finish chewing and swallowing before you put more food on your fork and if you're eating with others, talk a lot! That way your meal will last longer.

Put more energy into everything you do – walk faster, run up the stairs and walk up escalators, do any housework as vigorously as possible.

Your body can't store fitness so try to exercise as often, long and hard as you can manage comfortably. And choose activities that you enjoy – you're more likely to stick to exercise that you find fun or satisfying, rather than exercise you dread doing!

Eating out? Try and only have a two-course meal – a three-course meal is so much more than you'd eat for dinner at home anyway. Choose a fruit-based starter – such as melon – as one of the courses rather than having a calorie-laden dessert.

Eat before you go to a party – most party food oozes calories. Decline any offers of food politely, saying you've already eaten. There's no need to say why, either.

SNACK ATTACKS

50-CALORIE SNACKS:
(have two of these a day)
- 2 sticks celery, 1 medium carrot and 2tbsp low-fat natural yoghurt flavoured with mild curry powder
- 1 carton low-fat fruit yoghurt
- 150ml/6floz unsweetened fruit juice
- 1 selection from the 'fruit bowl'
- 150ml/¼pt skimmed milk and a dash of low-sugar Ribena
- 2tbsp raisins
- 3 bread sticks
- 1 Jaffa Cake

100 CALORIE SNACKS:
(have one a day in place of two 50-calorie snacks)
- 6 fresh or dried dates
- 2 high-fibre crispbreads with 1tsp peanut butter
- 1 mini pitta bread with Marmite or Vegemite and cucumber slices
- 1 slice toast with 1tsp jam or honey
- 2 high-fibre crispbreads and 25g/1oz houmous
- 1 toasted crumpet and a scraping of low-fat spread and 1tsp jam
- 2 Jaffa Cakes
- 3 chocolate fingers

If you're tempted to nibble on 'non-diet' foods, try this trick: clean your teeth or have a cup of Marmite. You won't want to eat after that.

If you feel like eating but it's not mealtime yet, find something else to do to fill in time – exercise to music, go for a walk or phone a friend.

Drinking a glass or two of cool water can help to keep hunger pangs at bay for a while as it can be easy to confuse thirst for hunger.

Writing down what you eat in a food diary can help, especially if you feel yourself starting to wander off the straight and narrow.

Weigh yourself no more frequently than once a week – on the same scales, wearing the same clothes (or none) and at the same time of day.

Eating very occasional high-calorie foods will not affect weight loss – but it will if you find yourself doing it frequently or on a regular basis.

Eat slowly, savouring every mouthful. If you don't rush, you'll be less tempted to overeat and less likely to suffer from indigestion.

Eat your meals off a smaller plate so your portions don't look miniscule compared to what you used to eat! It might sound silly, but it works!

Don't overcook your vegetables. If you steam your veggies you'll get more nutrients out of them, which will leave you feeling healthier and full of energy. Crunchier veggies will also take you longer to eat – another way to prevent you from eating too quickly and subsequently overeating.

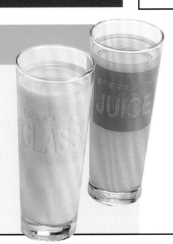

LIGHT MEALS (350 CALS)
All menus serve one, unless otherwise stated

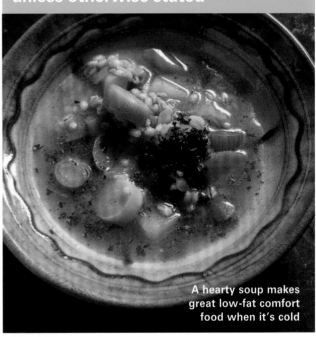

A hearty soup makes great low-fat comfort food when it's cold

BARLEY AND VEGETABLE SOUP (V) (SERVES 4)

1.4l/2½pt vegetable stock

1 bouquet garni

75g/3oz pearl barley

25g/1oz polyunsaturated margarine

3 carrots, peeled and sliced

3 celery sticks, washed and sliced

1 onion, peeled and chopped

225g/8oz mushrooms, peeled and roughly chopped

1tsp lemon juice

Bring the stock to the boil. Add the bouquet garni and pearl barley, and simmer for 45 minutes. Melt the margarine in a pan and cook the carrots, celery and onion until the onion is just softened. Add the cooked barley and the rest of the stock and cook gently for a further 10 minutes. Add the mushrooms and cook for another 5 minutes. Remove the bouquet garni, add the lemon juice and season with black pepper. Serve with a 50g/2oz wholemeal roll and 1 Mini Babybel Light. Finish with a portion of fruit.

CHEESY FRUIT POTATOES (V)

200g/7oz baking potato, scrubbed
(raw weight)

25g/1oz low-fat cottage cheese

25g/1oz raisins

25g/1oz dried apricots, chopped

Set the oven to 200°C/400°F/gas mark 6. Prick the potato and bake it for 1-1½ hours. Mix the other ingredients together and season. Slit the potato almost in half and spoon in the filling. Finish with a 115g/4oz pot of low-fat yoghurt.

PITTA BREAD PIZZA (V)

1 wholemeal pitta bread

150g can baked beans in tomato sauce

25g/1oz low-fat Cheddar or
Cheshire cheese

Warm the pitta under a grill and heat the beans in a saucepan. Pile the beans onto the pitta and crumble the cheese over the top. Grill until the cheese melts and starts to bubble. Finish with a portion of fruit.

SARDINE SANDWICHES

2 medium slices from a large wholemeal loaf

2tsp low-fat spread

2 sardines in tomato sauce

Cucumber slices

Spread the bread with the low-fat spread, fill with the sardines and cucumber slices. Follow with a 70g pot of Marks & Spencer Count On Us… Chocolate Mousse.

PASTRAMI ROLL

1 granary roll

2tsp low-fat spread

50g/2oz pastrami

Sliced gherkins and mustard (optional)

Split the roll and spread with the low-fat spread. Fill with pastrami and gherkins and add mustard, if desired. Finish with a portion of fruit and 115g/4oz pot of low-fat yoghurt.

PITTA AND VEG DIP (V)

1 wholemeal pitta bread

Sticks of assorted raw vegetables

3tbsp tzatziki

Lightly toast the pitta bread and cut it into strips. Serve with the raw vegetable sticks and the tzatziki. Finish with a 50g packet of ready-to-eat apricots.

PASTA SALAD

115g/4oz cooked brown rice

50g/2oz tuna in brine, drained
and flaked

Diced cucumber

1 red pepper, deseeded and diced

75g/3oz black grapes, halved

Lemon juice to taste

Garlic to taste

Toss all the ingredients in lemon juice flavoured with crushed garlic and freshly ground pepper. Serve the salad with 2 bread sticks. Finish with a portion of fruit.

MAIN MEALS (400 CALS) All menus serve one, unless otherwise stated

MEATY GOULASH (SERVES 4)

25g/1oz plain flour

Pinch of mustard powder

1tbsp paprika

565g/1¼lb chicken, skinned and cubed

2tbsp sunflower oil

2 onions, sliced into rings

1 green and 1 red pepper, deseeded and sliced

400g can chopped tomatoes

600ml/1pt vegetables stock

150ml/5floz low-fat natural yoghurt

Set the oven to 160°C/325°F/gas mark 3. Mix together the flour, mustard and paprika and toss the chicken in the mixture. Heat the oil in a pan and fry the chicken until brown. Transfer to a casserole dish. Fry the onions and peppers, add to the dish with the tomatoes and stock. Cook in the oven for 1-1¼ hours. Spoon over the yoghurt and serve with 115g/4oz boiled rice. Finish with a portion of fruit.

LAMB KEBABS (SERVES 4)

5tbsp lemon juice

5tbsp light soy sauce

1 clove garlic, peeled and crushed

450g/1lb lean lamb in 3.75cm/1½in cubes

8 small or cherry tomatoes

12 button or small mushrooms, trimmed

1 green pepper, deseeded and cut into cubes

1 onion, cut into wedges

½ cabbage, grated

4 carrots, peeled and grated

2 apples, cored (not peeled) and diced

Mix together the lemon juice, soy sauce and garlic. Marinate the meat in the mixture for at least 2 hours. Thread the meat, tomatoes, mushrooms, peppers and onions onto skewers. Cook the kebabs under a hot grill, turning and basting with the marinade, until the meat is tender. Heat and serve the leftover marinade with the kebabs. Mix together the remaining

ingredients and pile in a dish with the kebabs on top. Serve with a warmed wholemeal pitta. Finish with a large slice of melon.

SUNDAY ROAST

75g/3oz lean roast meat eg chicken or beef

200g/7oz medium jacket potato (raw weight)

Assorted unlimited vegetables

Serve the roast meat with the jacket potato and vegetables. Finish with 50g/2oz sorbet.

CURRIED FISH (SERVES 4)

450g/1lb potatoes, peeled and cut into chunks

1tbsp sunflower oil

1 onion, peeled and chopped

2 cloves of garlic, peeled and crushed

15g/½oz fresh ginger root, chopped

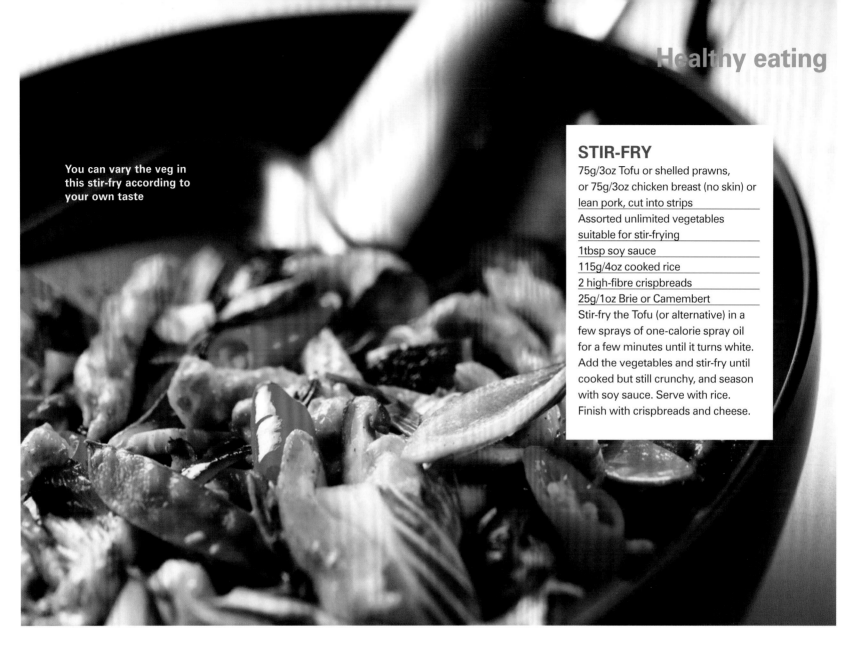

You can vary the veg in this stir-fry according to your own taste

STIR-FRY

75g/3oz Tofu or shelled prawns, or 75g/3oz chicken breast (no skin) or lean pork, cut into strips

Assorted unlimited vegetables suitable for stir-frying

1tbsp soy sauce

115g/4oz cooked rice

2 high-fibre crispbreads

25g/1oz Brie or Camembert

Stir-fry the Tofu (or alternative) in a few sprays of one-calorie spray oil for a few minutes until it turns white. Add the vegetables and stir-fry until cooked but still crunchy, and season with soy sauce. Serve with rice. Finish with crispbreads and cheese.

Curry powder to taste

450g/1lb white fish fillet, skinned and cut into 2.5cm/1in pieces

1 red pepper, deseeded and sliced

400g can chopped tomatoes

Parboil the potatoes for 5 minutes. Heat the oil in a pan and lightly cook the onion. Add the garlic, ginger and curry powder and cook for 1 minute. Add the fish, peppers, potatoes and tomatoes. Bring to the boil, then cover and simmer for 15 minutes. Serve with 115g/ 4oz boiled rice. Finish with a portion of fruit.

PASTA BOLOGNESE

75g/3oz extra lean mince

1 onion, chopped

200g can chopped tomatoes

75g/3oz mushrooms, wiped and chopped

Mixed herbs

150g/5oz cooked spaghetti

Assorted unlimited vegetables

Dry-fry the mince in a nonstick pan until it browns. Add the onion and cook until softened. Add the tomatoes, mushrooms and herbs. Simmer for 20 minutes. Serve with the spaghetti and vegetables. Finish with 115g/ 4oz fruit salad and 2tbsp fat-free fromage frais.

MEAT OR FISH PIE

75g/3oz extra lean mince or 105g can pink salmon

1 onion, chopped

200g can chopped tomatoes

150g/5oz cooked potato, mashed (made with milk from daily allowance)

Dry-fry the meat or fish with the onion. Stir in the tomatoes and simmer until the meat or fish is cooked. Season. Tip into a heatproof dish, top with the potato and brown under the grill. Finish with 1 Jordans Frusli bar.

What shape are you?

Tick the boxes at the end of the statements that you think match your body shape most closely

Do you:
A: gain weight on your torso while your arms and legs stay slim? ☐
B: put on weight on your hips and bottom? ☐
C: tend to put weight on all over? ☐

Are you:
A: larger around your waist and tummy? ☐
B: smaller up top and bigger below? ☐
C: carrying extra weight pretty evenly all over your body? ☐

When you go shopping for clothes are you:
A: conscious of your protruding stomach? ☐
B: conscious of your large bottom and hips? ☐
C: conscious of your flabby legs and arms? ☐

Do you put on weight:
A: around your middle and have 'love handles'? ☐
B: on your bum and on your thighs? ☐
C: all over, especially on your arms and at the tops of your legs? ☐

Do you want to:
A: lose weight and tone up your middle? ☐
B: lose weight all over and tone up your hips and thighs? ☐
C: lose weight all over and increase your general muscle tone? ☐

What's your body shape?

Are you an apple, pear or hourglass? Whatever your body shape, we've designed the perfect diet...

DIET: JUDITH WILLS; PHOTOGRAPHY: ANDREW SYDENHAM/BIG PICTURES

Diet plans for you

If you ticked mostly As, you're an Apple
You have a thicker torso and store excess weight around your stomach and back. Your legs and arms tend to remain slim.
Follow our apple-shapes diet.

If you ticked mostly Bs, you're a Pear
You have a smaller chest with wider hips, thighs and bottom. The right exercise programme can make you look more in proportion.
Follow our pear-shapes diet.

If you ticked mostly Cs, you're an Hourglass
You tend to put on weight evenly, and all over. This can make you look curvy but lacking in overall tone and shape.
Try following our hourglass-shapes diet.

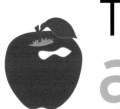

The diet for
apple shapes

Thick waist and 'baby bulge'? Give our tailor-made health plan a whirl...

The classic apple shape is a big waist and stomach; slim arms and legs. This shape is linked to a higher risk of heart disease – on the up in women. Concentrating on eating foods low on the GI Index is a good way to lose weight from those problem areas. The GI measures how fast carbohydrate foods are absorbed. Low GI foods such as pulses, veg, some fruits, yoghurt and wholegrains help to keep blood sugar levels constant and keep you full for longer. So our apple shape diet will focus on these. You can also chomp on nuts and seeds which give vital 'good' fats, and lean protein foods, all of which help to balance out any higher GI foods – such as sugar, chocolate, cakes and processed foods you might have in a meal.

The diet also has foods which help to minimise your middle in other ways, such as plenty of diuretic foods to help control any fluid retention. Also, the foods have plenty of fibre so you don't have to worry about constipation.

Like any diet, you'll need to combine it with regular exercise (this means 30 mins, two to three times a week) for it to work. But, when you do, your tum will be reduced fast – and you won't be left feeling hungry, either.

Here's what to do:

Follow the basic diet and have your milk and fruit allowances, and pick a *Breakfast*, *Lunch* and *Dinner* each day from the choices. Then, depending on how much weight you have to lose, pick your *Snacks*, and check out the unlimited items. Any fruit or milk in meals are extra to your allowance (unless stated otherwise). Spread your meals and snacks out through the day – important for keeping blood-sugar stable – and don't skip meals – it'll work against you in the long run.

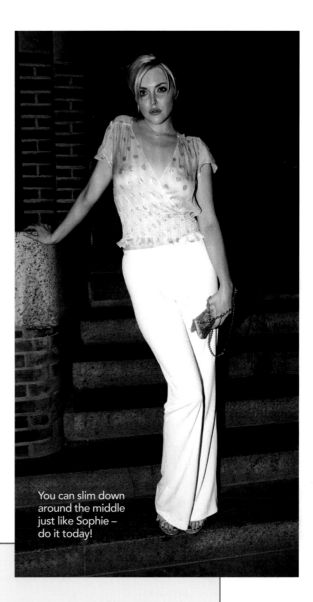

You can slim down around the middle just like Sophie – do it today!

Your snack allowance

★ **If you have less than 1st to lose,** follow the basic diet and have ONE snack each day from the 125-calorie *Snacks* list. Have your 100-calorie milk allowance as well as any milk mentioned in the recipes (unless stated otherwise), to total 1,250 cals each day.

★ **If you have 1st to 3st to lose,** follow the basic diet and have either TWO snacks a day from the 125-cal *Snacks* list; OR ONE snack a day from the 250-cal *Snacks* list, plus your milk allowance, to bring your total daily cals to 1,500.

★ **If you have over 3st to lose,** follow the basic diet and have EITHER FOUR snacks a day from the 125-cal *Snacks* list; OR TWO snacks a day from the 250-cal *Snacks* list; OR TWO 125-calorie snacks and ONE 250-calorie snack. Plus have your 100-calorie milk allowance, to total 1,750 calories a day.

apple shapes

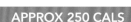

YOUR DAILY MILK ALLOWANCE

Each day have 200ml/7floz skimmed milk for use in hot drinks, or on its own. This is extra to any milk used in the meal choices.

DAILY FRUIT ALLOWANCE

Pick one portion of fruit from this list each day. Vary your choices so you don't miss essential nutrients. These fruits are low on the GI scale:

∗1 medium orange, pear, apple or peach

∗ ½ grapefruit

∗ 2 plums

∗ 1 handful fresh cherries

∗ 4 whole ready-to-eat dried apricots

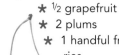

UNLIMITED ITEMS

Water, mineral water, very weak regular tea, herbal tea, redbush tea (or rooibos), green tea, freshly-squeezed lemon or lime juice, fresh or dried herbs and spices, oil-free French dressing, green salad items, cucumber, celery and dark leafy green vegetables.

Nibble on your fruit allowance through the day to keep blood-sugar levels even and cravings at bay

APPROX 250 CALS

Breakfasts

● **Fruity yoghurt** 50ml/ ¼ pot low-fat natural bio-yoghurt topped with 4 chopped, dried, ready-to-eat apricots; 1 small chopped apple; and 1 level dsp chopped, mixed nuts.

● **Bread 'n' jam** 1 x 30g slice wholemeal bread with 1tsp low-fat spread and reduced-sugar jam or marmalade; ½ pink grapefruit; 200ml pot Müllerlight yoghurt.

● **Fruit muesli** 175ml/6floz low-fat natural bio-yoghurt; 100g/3½oz raspberries or strawberries (fresh) and 1 handful unsweetened muesli with 1 level tsp caster sugar.

● **Banana milkshake** Blend 200ml/7floz semi-skimmed milk with 1 medium banana.

● **Fruity muesli** 60g/2¼oz no-added-sugar muesli with skimmed milk from allowance to cover, and 1 chopped apple or peach.

● **Cereal filler** 2 Shredded Wheat with 100ml/4floz skimmed milk (not allowance); 2 plums.

● **Sticky wheatgerm** Blend 2tsp runny honey and 1tsp wheatgerm in an electric mixer; serve with 1 handful cherries.

● **Cereal and juice** 2 Weetabix with skimmed milk (from allowance) to cover; and 1 level tsp caster sugar; 1 orange.

Lunches

APPROX 350 CALS

● **Tuna and bean salad** Mix 100g/3½oz can tuna in oil, drained, with 4 heaped tbsp cooked, brown basmati rice; 60g/ 2¼oz canned, rinsed cannellini beans; 2 spring onions, chopped; 1 ripe tomato, chopped; fresh basil. Toss in 1tbsp low-fat French dressing.

● **Waldorf salad** Chop 1 small red, dessert apple and 2 small sticks celery and mix with 125g/4½oz cooked, diced, chicken breast; 4 walnut halves, crumbled; 1dsp reduced-calorie mayonnaise mixed with 1tbsp bio-yoghurt, a little lemon juice and seasoning. Serve with 1 slice dark rye bread from a small ready-sliced loaf.

● **Chilli salmon salad** Poach (or microwave on medium) 100g/3¼oz salmon fillet for 2 minutes. Flake the fish and mix with 4tbsp cooked, whole-wheat pasta shapes; 1 handful fresh beansprouts; strips of cucumber, spring onion and carrot; plus some fresh coriander leaves and finely-chopped fresh chilli. Dress with 1tbsp oil-free French dressing.

● **Avocado, prawn salad** Gently combine ½ small sliced avocado with 100g/ 3oz peeled

Snacks

APPROX 125 CALS

● 1 small banana and 4 dried apricots.
● 125g pot low-fat fruit flavour bio-yoghurt; plus 6 almonds.
● 1 level tbsp peanut butter on 1 rice cake.
● 2 dark rye Ryvitas with 1tbsp low-fat soft cheese.
● 1tsp low-fat spread and Marmite on 1 medium slice wholemeal bread.
● 100g/3½oz pot Shape low-fat fruit flavour fromage frais with 1 traditional oatcake.
● 25g trail mix.
● 2 traditional oatcakes topped with 1tbsp any low-fat savoury ready-made dip.
● 40g/1½oz slice rich, fruit cake.
● 30g/1oz slice date and walnut loaf.

prawns; 3tbsp cooked, brown basmati rice or buckwheat; 1 large chopped tomato; and thinly-sliced little gem lettuce hearts. Add 2tbsp oil-free French dressing.

● **Pitta and houmous** Fill a wholewheat pitta with 2tbsp low-fat houmous – thinned with a little oil-free French dressing – and chopped tomato, cucumber, red onion and lettuce. Plus 1 apple.

● **Crudités and dips** Serve 100ml/4floz ready-made tzatziki and 50ml/2floz ready-made guacamole with a large selection of fresh fruit and vegetable crudités (go for slices of apple, celery, chicory, carrot and peppers) and 1 wholewheat pitta bread, cut into dipping strips.

● **Soup and bread** 300ml/¹⁄₂pt fresh deli counter mixed bean or lentil and vegetable soup served with 1 large slice (40g/1¹⁄₂oz) wholemeal bread. Plus 5 ready-to-eat dried apricot halves.

● **Baked beans on toast** 200/7oz baked beans in tomato sauce poured on to 1 large slice (40g/1¹⁄₂oz) wholegrain toast spread with 2tsp low-fat spread. Plus 1 kiwi fruit.

Snacks

APPROX 250 CALS

● 250ml low-fat bio-yoghurt blended with 1 whole, peeled, stoned, peach; 50ml/2floz orange juice and 2tsp runny honey.
● Fill 1 wholemeal pitta with 1tbsp salsa; 75g/3oz lean, cooked, chopped chicken, plus salad.
● 2 thin slices wholemeal bread with 2tsp low-fat spread and 1tbsp medium-fat soft cheese to fill.
● 3 traditional oatcakes with 25g/1oz reduced-fat Cheddar and 1dsp pickle.
● Fill 1 wholemeal pitta with 1tbsp reduced-fat houmous and some chopped salad.

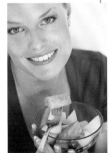

Dinners

APPROX 400 CALS

● **Moroccan casserole** Heat 1dsp olive oil in a non-stick pan. Add 150g/5oz boneless, skinless chicken breast portion; 1 small onion, sliced and browned. Add 65g/2¹⁄₂oz canned, drained chickpeas; 200g/7oz chopped, canned tomatoes; 1tsp ground cumin; 1tsp harissa paste. Simmer for 25 minutes or until the chicken is cooked. Serve on 3tbsp cooked bulgar wheat, garnished with 1dsp flaked almonds. Eat with green veg.

● **Bacon and bean compote** Cook 150g/5oz-(raw weight) new potatoes then drain, dice and keep warm. Meanwhile, cook 100g/3¹⁄₂oz fresh or frozen green or broad beans, drain and keep warm. Grill 2 x 25g/1oz slices extra-lean back bacon then crumble while warm. Mix the ingredients with 1dsp freshly-chopped parsley and 1dsp freshly-chopped mint and 1–2tbsp oil-free French dressing. Serve immediately with a large, mixed side salad.

● **Cod with chilli lentils** Simmer 40g/1¹⁄₂oz dried puy or brown lentils for 30 minutes, until tender. Drain and add 1 small, finely-chopped jalapeno chilli; 1 shallot, chopped; 100g/ 3¹⁄₂oz canned, chopped tomatoes; and salt and black pepper to taste. Simmer for 10 minutes. Meanwhile microwave, grill or bake 1 x 200g/7oz cod fillet. Serve fish on top of the lentils with steamed broccoli or spinach.

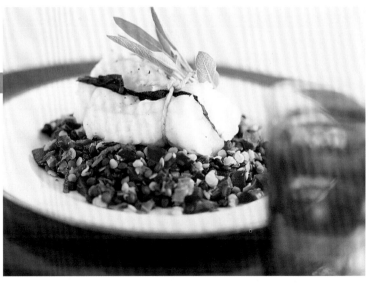

● **Turkey and noodle stir-fry** Cook 40g/1¹⁄₂oz wholewheat noodles according to instructions. Meanwhile, in a non-stick pan, with 1dsp groundnut oil, stir-fry 125g/4¹⁄₂oz fresh turkey breast, sliced into strips; plus a selection of sliced, fresh veg (go for carrots, courgettes, green beans, mangetout) and 1dsp each of soya sauce and black-bean sauce. Serve on the noodles.

● **Veggie curry:** Chop a 350g/12oz selection of veg (go for cauliflower, carrots, squash, aubergine, onion) and simmer in 150ml/¹⁄₄pt Patak's Dopiaza curry sauce, until tender. Stir in 100g/3¹⁄₂oz baby spinach leaves and serve on top of 4tbsp cooked, brown, basmati rice with a dollop of low-fat bio-yoghurt; garnish with some diced cucumber.
● **Meat and plenty of veg** Three small slices lean roast beef or pork served with 150g/5oz baked sweet potato, topped with 1tsp butter. Serve with cooked green beans, courgettes and peas, fat-skimmed gravy and 1tsp relish of your choice.

The diet for **pear shapes**

The perfect plan for those who have 'stubborn' bums 'n' tums

Hip and thigh fat won't always disappear as easily as fat around the middle, so, if you have a pear-shaped body, you'll need to really target those parts to shift the weight.

But don't worry, if you love fruit, veg, potatoes, bread, pasta, rice, Indian, Chinese and meals from the Med – and you can happily get by without eating huge quantities of meat – then a low-fat diet is the

one for you.

Research shows that if weight is lost steadily, it's most likely to stay off for good. And the low-fat way really is a good, steady route to shedding pounds, unlike more drastic low-carb or high-protein diets.

Couple our delicious low-fat diet with regular lower body and aerobic exercise and you can reshape your body and unveil the new, curvy you.

Showing off her best assets – curvaceous Kate has got the look

Here's what to do

Follow the basic diet by having your milk and fruit allowances each day, and pick a *Breakfast*, *Lunch* and *Dinner* every day from the choices that we have provided for you. Check out the list of other items you can enjoy in unlimited amounts, too, and, depending on how much weight you want to lose, pick one or more *Snacks* each day . You can have any fruit or milk stated within each of the individual meal suggestions in addition to your daily milk and fruit allowances. Start your new diet today, and look forward to a slim and healthy new you!

YOUR DAILY MILK ALLOWANCE

Each day have 200ml/7floz skimmed milk for hot drinks or on its own. This is extra to any milk used in the meal choices.

DAILY FRUIT ALLOWANCE

Pick one fruit portion from this list and vary your choices so you don't miss out on any nutrients.

* 1 apple, pear, orange, peach, nectarine or small banana.
* 2 clementines or satsumas, 2 fresh apricots, 2 plums, or 2 kiwi fruit.
* 75g/3oz grapes or 100g/3½oz cherries.
* 1 slice melon, ½ grapefruit, or 2 rings pineapple.
* Medium bowl of berries such as strawberries.

UNLIMITED ITEMS

Water, mineral water, very weak regular tea, herbal tea, fruit teas, green tea, white tea redbush tea (also called rooibos), freshly-squeezed lemon or lime juice, fresh or dried herbs and spices, oil-free French dressing, green salad items, celery, cucumber and dark green veggies such as spinach, cabbage and broccoli.

Your snack allowance

* **Up to 1st to lose;** follow the basic diet and have ONE 125-cal snack a day from the *Snacks* list, plus your milk and fruit allowances: total 1,250 cals a day.
* **1st to 3st to lose;** follow the diet and have either TWO 125-cal snacks OR ONE 250-cal snack a day, plus your milk and fruit: total 1,500 cals a day.
* **Over 3st to lose;** follow the diet and have EITHER FOUR 125-cal snacks a day; OR TWO 250-cal snacks a day; OR TWO 125-cal snacks and ONE 250-cal snack: total 1,750 cals a day.

Breakfasts

APPROX 250 CALS

● **Fruity yoghurt** 200g/ 7oz pot Müllerlight yoghurt; 1 large banana; ½ pink grapefruit with 1tsp caster sugar.

● **Weetabix and banana** 2 Weetabix with 1tsp caster sugar, skimmed milk to cover. Plus 1 medium banana.

● **Cereal and fruit** 40g/ 1½oz Fruit 'n' Fibre with skimmed milk (extra to allowance). 1 medium slice melon and 100ml/ 3½floz unsweetened juice.

● **Cereal and toast** 5g/1oz bran-flakes with skimmed milk to cover; 1 medium slice toast with 1tsp low-fat spread and 1tsp jam or marmalade; 100ml/3½floz juice.

● **Yoghurt filler** 125g pot low-fat bio yoghurt topped with 1tbsp muesli, 2 chopped dates. Plus 1 small banana.

● **Special K plus!** 40g/ 1½oz Special K Red Berries with skimmed milk to cover; 1 thin slice toast, with 1tsp low-fat spread and 1tsp honey.

● **Toast and yoghurt** 2 medium slices toast, 2tsp low-fat spread and 2tsp jam; 125g pot diet yoghurt.

It's a low-fat plan with around 25% of cals from fat – but you won't lose out on essential oils

Lunches

APPROX 350 CALS

● **Beans on toast** 200g/ 7oz baked beans on 1 medium slice wholemeal toast with 1tsp low-fat spread. Plus 1 kiwi fruit or nectarine and 125g/4½oz Shape fromage frais.

● **Cheesy bean potato** 250g/9oz baked potato with 100g/3½oz baked beans and 2 slices light cheese on top.

● **Basic sandwich** Fill 2 medium slices wholemeal bread with 1 level tbsp Hellmann's Dijonnaise and 100g/3½oz drained tuna in springwater or brine, or wafer-thin ham, with lettuce, tomato and cucumber. Plus 1 apple.

● **Prawn sandwich** Fill 2 medium slices wholemeal bread with 1tbsp Hellmann's Reduced-calorie 1000 Island sauce, 100g/3½oz peeled prawns and lettuce. Plus 2 plums.

● **Chicken pitta** Fill 1 wholemeal pitta bread with 100g/3½oz lean chicken, 2tbsp reduced-cal coleslaw and 50g/2oz halved cherry tomatoes. Plus 50g/2oz fresh, grapes or cherries.

● **Greek wrap** Fill 1 wholemeal pitta bread or tortilla wrap with 40g/1½oz reduced-fat houmous, and some chopped, crisp salad, plus 5 halved cherry tomatoes.

● **Sandwich or wrap** Pre-packed, shop-bought, containing around 300 calories and 10g fat. Plus 1 apple.

● **Soup** Shop-bought at around 200 calories and 6g fat; 1 wholemeal roll with 1tsp low-fat spread. Plus 125g pot Shape fromage frais.
● **Feta salad** Prepare some chopped lettuce, cucumber, tomato chunks, chopped red onion, sliced red pepper, 2 halved black olives (optional) and 40g/ 1½oz feta cheese. Toss in a bowl and drizzle over oil-free French dressing; serve with 1 medium roll. Plus 1 papaya or 1 pear.

● **Chicken tikka salad** Mix together 100g/3½oz shop-bought chicken tikka slices with a large mixed salad including watercress or rocket, halved cherry tomatoes, red and yellow pepper, and chopped onion. Toss in a bowl, drizzle over oil-free French dressing and serve with 1 medium slice bread with 1tsp low-fat spread. Plus 125g pot Shape fromage frais.

● **Handy lunchbox** 1 Boots Shapers Prawn Cocktail Pasta, or similar containing around 300 calories and 10g fat. Plus 1 peach or 1 nectarine.

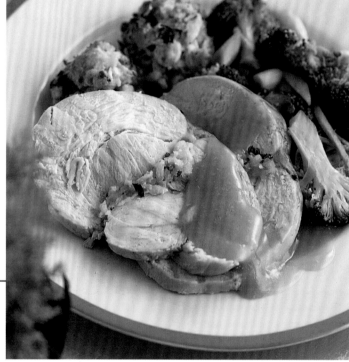

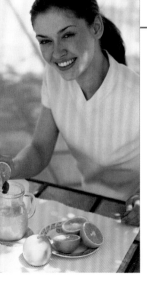

Dinners

APPROX 400 CALS

● **Fish pie** 1 portion frozen cod in parsley sauce; 150g/5oz potatoes (raw weight), mashed with 2tsp low-fat spread and skimmed milk; 100g/3½oz peas and 100g/3½oz broccoli.

● **Ready meal** Your choice of meal, served with a side salad or a selection of steamed, fresh veggies.

● **Meat and veg** 125g/ 4½oz roast beef or pork (all visible fat removed); a selection of your choice of fresh vegetables; 100g/ 3½oz new potatoes (raw weight); with 2tbsp fat-skimmed gravy and 1dsp relish of your choice.

● **Tuna grill** Grill a 150g/ 5oz fresh tuna steak for 2 mins each side or to taste. Meanwhile, chop 2 stoned black olives and 1 large spring onion, then stir into 3tbsp ready-made tomato pasta sauce and heat. Serve with a few freshly-chopped basil leaves and 50g/2oz (dry weight) pasta, cooked according to the pack instructions. Serve with 100g/3½oz green beans.

(continued next page)

pear shapes

● **Cod with bacon sauce and vegetables**
Preheat oven to 200°C/400°F/gas mark 6. Place 200g/7oz cod fillet or steak on a non-stick baking tray and top with 3tbsp Loyd Grossman Smoky Bacon Pasta Sauce and sprinkle over 1 medium tomato, roughly chopped. Bake for 20 minutes, or until cooked through. Serve the fish with 100g/3½oz new potatoes (raw weight); and 100g/3½oz broccoli or green beans.

● **Veggie stir-fry** Take 150g/5oz Quorn pieces and stir-fry in 1dsp sesame oil with a large selection of thinly-sliced vegetables added to the wok (go for carrots, red peppers, courgettes, mangetout or broccoli). Add 2tbsp vegetable stock, 1tbsp hoisin sauce, and 1tsp soya sauce towards the end of the cooking time. Serve on top of 50g/2oz (dry weight), noodles or 4tbsp boiled rice, cooked according to the pack instructions.

● **Chicken brochette** Cut 150g/5oz chicken fillet into bite-size pieces and marinate for 1 to 2 hours in 2tbsp low-fat yoghurt, mixed with 1tsp mild curry powder. Thread onto a kebab stick and grill for 10 mins, turning once. Serve with 4tbsp boiled rice and a tomato and cucumber salad. Follow with 200g/7oz pot Müllerlight yoghurt.

● **Spaghetti marinara** Cook 75g/3oz (dry weight) spaghetti, according to the pack instructions. Meanwhile, simmer 4tbsp Dolmio Original Sauce with 100g/3½oz (frozen weight) mixed, defrosted seafood for 10 minutes. Pour the sauce over the cooked spaghetti and top with 1 level dsp grated Parmesan. Serve with a large mixed side salad, with fresh crisp lettuce, chopped pepper and onion tossed in oil-free French dressing.

● **Chicken and potato**
Serve 150g/5oz chicken breast, grilled then skinned, with 250g/9oz baked potato, 1tsp butter or 2 tsp low-fat spread, and a selection of fresh, cooked vegetables.

● **Yogurt mustard salmon and mange tout** Serve 100g/3½oz grilled salmon steak or fillet, with 100g/ 3½oz (raw weight) cooked, new potatoes and 60g/2¼oz mangetout. Dress salmon with sauce made by mixing 1 level tbsp Hellmann's Dijonnaise with 1 level tbsp low-fat bio yoghurt and a squeeze of lemon juice. Plus 1 banana.

Snacks

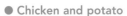

APPROX 125 CALS

● 1 medium slice bread with 1tsp low-fat spread and Marmite. Plus 1 plum.
● 3 Dark Rye Ryvitas with 100g/3½oz low-fat cottage cheese on top and some cherry tomatoes.
● 30g/1¼oz bag pretzels.
● 1 medium banana; 2 dried apricots.
● 3 fat-free crackers with 30g/1¼oz low-fat soft cheese and a spreading of 1tbsp sweet pickle.
● 1 medium slice wholemeal bread; with 1 x 22.5g Dairylea Triangle; 1 tomato.
● 1 pot Low-Fat Ambrosia Devon Custard.
● 1 mini wholemeal pitta bread; 1 level tbsp low-fat soft cheese; 1 finely-sliced tomato.
● 1 Boots Shapers Strawberry Delight Dessert.
● 2 rice cakes; 4tsp reduced-sugar jam.
● 30g/1¼oz bag sweet popcorn.

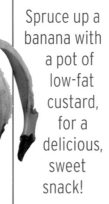

Spruce up a banana with a pot of low-fat custard, for a delicious, sweet snack!

Snacks

APPROX 250 CALS

● 200g/7oz pot Müllerice.
● 125g/4½oz Shape Greek-style Yoghurt; plus 1 large banana.
● 400g/14oz Sainsbury's Be Good To Yourself soup; plus 1 medium slice wholemeal bread.
● 1 Boots Shapers Tuna Pasta Salad.
● 1 pot Low-Fat Ambrosia Custard mixed with 1 medium sliced banana.
● 2 medium slices wholemeal bread filled with 50g/2oz wafer-thin ham and salad. Plus a spreading of 2tsp reduced-cal mayo.

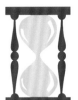

The diet for hourglass shapes

Does your weight gain go all over, instead of plumping up one area? Then we've designed this healthy-eating plan just for you...

Women with a shape termed as 'hourglass' don't usually need to go on a super-strict diet to lose weight – if they just swap to a healthier eating plan, they should find it comes off quite well. Sound like you? Then try this balanced plan for great results. It'll give you plenty to eat and we've included delicious desserts and snacks so you don't have to deny yourself.

By cutting out many of the fatty foods and drinks that people often eat lots of without realising – things like sugary drinks, pastry products, high-fat cheeses and full-fat sauces – it's easy to cut enough calories for good weight loss.

This plan lets you pick your meals, but vary your choices for good health. They're quick and easy – and tasty and filling, too!

Here's what to do

Follow the basic diet by having your daily milk and fruit allowances and pick a *Breakfast*, *Lunch* and *Dinner* every day from the choices we've provided. Check out the list of other items you can enjoy in unlimited amounts, too, and, depending on how much weight you want to lose, pick one or more *Snacks* each day. Any fruit or milk stated used within the individual meal suggestions is in addition to your daily milk and fruit allowances. Start today for a slim and healthy new you!

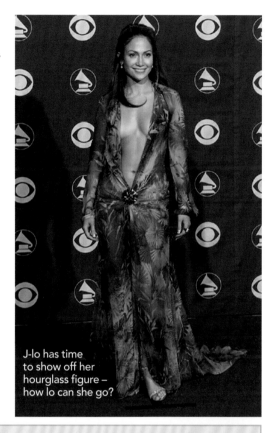

J-lo has time to show off her hourglass figure – how lo can she go?

YOUR DAILY MILK ALLOWANCE

Each day have 200ml skimmed milk for use in hot drinks, or on its own. This is extra to any milk used in the meal choices.

YOUR DAILY FRUIT ALLOWANCE

Pick one portion of fruit from this list every day. Vary your choices as much as possible so you don't miss out on any essential nutrients:

* 1 apple, pear, orange, peach, or small banana.
* 2 satsumas, 2 plums, 2 kiwi fruit, 2 fresh apricots.

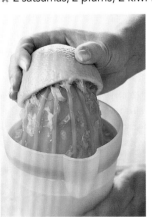

* 75g/3oz grapes or 100g/3½oz cherries.
* ½ grapefruit, 2 rings pineapple or 1 slice melon.
* Medium bowl of berries such as strawberries, raspberries or loganberries.

UNLIMITED ITEMS

Water, mineral water, very weak regular tea, herbal tea, green tea, redbush tea (also called rooibos), freshly-squeezed lemon or lime juice, fresh or dried herbs and spices, oil-free French dressing, green salad, celery, cucumber and leafy green veg.

Fruits are a great choice of natural sugars to help keep you off the chocs!

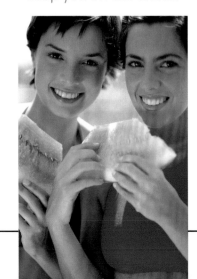

Your snack allowance

* **If you have less than 1st to lose,** follow the basic diet and have ONE snack each day from the 125-cal *Snacks* list, plus your 100-cal milk allowance, to total 1,250 cals each day.
* **If you have 1st to 3st to lose,** follow the basic diet and have either TWO snacks a day from the 125-cal *Snacks* list; OR ONE snack a day from the 250-cal *Snacks* list, and your milk allowance, to bring your total daily cals to 1,500.
* **If you have over 3st to lose,** follow the basic diet and have EITHER FOUR snacks a day from the 125-cal *Snacks* list; OR TWO snacks a day from the 250-cal *Snacks* list; OR TWO 125-calorie snacks and ONE 250-calorie snack. This will bring your total daily calories to approximately 1,750.

hourglass shapes

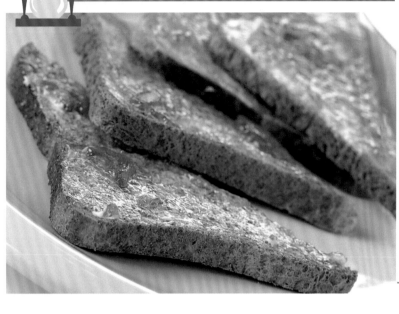

Breakfasts

● **Egg on toast** 1 boiled egg on 1 medium slice wholemeal toast with 2tsp low-fat spread; 150ml/ ¼pt orange juice.

● **Fruity muesli** 50g/2oz muesli with skimmed milk to cover, sprinkled with a few halved grapes.

● **Fruit and yoghurt** 200ml/7floz low-fat bio yoghurt with 150g/5oz berry fruits and 1tsp honey; 1 level tsp sunflower seeds.

● **Cereal** 2 Weetabix with skimmed milk to cover, and 1tsp caster sugar.

● **Fruity cereal** 40g/1½oz Kellogg's Special K Red Berries with skimmed milk to cover. Plus 1 banana.

● **Toast topper** 1 medium slice wholemeal toast with 1tsp low-fat spread and 1tsp Marmite, or 1tsp reduced-sugar jam, or 1tsp marmalade.

● **Bacon sarnie** 2 slices grilled extra-lean back bacon in 2 thin slices wholemeal bread; with 1tsp low-fat spread and 2tsp brown sauce.

● **Beans on toast** 200g/ 7oz baked beans on 1 medium slice wholemeal toast with 1tsp low-fat spread.

Lunches

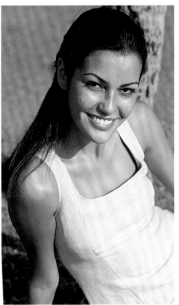

● **Mozzarella bap** Fill 1 wholemeal bap with salad and 40g/1½oz half-fat mozzarella cheese and spread on 2tsp Hellmann's Light Mayonnaise. Plus 1 Shape Low-fat Fromage Frais with some grapes.

● **Salad Niçoise** Drain a 200g can tuna in brine, with 1 sliced boiled egg; 100g/3½oz cooked, diced new potatoes; 1 sliced tomato; 1 sliced little gem lettuce; 2 halved black olives; and oil-free French dressing. Plus 1 peach.

● **Prawn and pasta salad** Mix 50g/2oz (dry weight) cooked pasta with 75g/ 3oz cooked, peeled prawns; 4 halved cherry tomatoes; 2 chopped spring onions and chopped cucumber. Toss in 1tbsp Hellmann's Reduced-calorie 1000 Island Dressing mixed with 1tbsp low-fat bio yoghurt.

● **Avocado salad** Peel and slice half a ripe avocado and toss with mixed baby salad leaves and rocket. Add ½ a sliced pepper, 1tsp pine nuts, and oil-free French dressing. Serve with 1 Ryvita Dark Rye.

● **Prepack sandwich** Up to 300 calories. Plus 1 apple.

● **Any ready-made salad** Up to 350 calories.

● **Nibbles and dip** 100g/ 3½oz low-fat ready-made savoury dip, served with a selection of vegetable crudités (go for pepper, carrot, celery and chicory); 6 mini breadsticks; and 1 wholemeal pitta bread, cut into strips.

● **Egg and cress salad** Quarter 2 boiled eggs and place in a bowl with 1 handful watercress; 1 handful halved cherry tomatoes; 3 chopped radishes; and 1-2 sliced spring onions. Drizzle with oil-free French dressing and serve with 1 slice medium wholemeal bread spread with 2tsp low-fat spread. Plus 1 pear.

● **Cheesy ciabatta** Cut 1 thick slice ciabatta bread and brush with 2tsp olive oil. Top with 40g/ 1½oz sliced goat's cheese and 1 sliced tomato. Grill until the cheese is bubbling.

● **Open salmon sandwich** 1 slice dark rye bread (pumpernickel) from a small, ready-sliced loaf, with 2tsp low-fat spread, topped with 65g/2½oz smoked salmon; lemon juice; black pepper; and chopped cucumber. 1 Shape Low-fat Fruit Yoghurt; plus 1 plum.

Dinners

APPROX 400 CALS

● **Turkey stir-fry** Slice 125g/4½oz fresh turkey breast and stir-fry for 1-2 minutes in 1tsp sesame oil with 75g/3oz chopped broccoli and 1 medium carrot, cut into strips. Add 1 sachet Blue Dragon Oyster & Spring Onion Sauce and heat for 1 minute while stirring. Serve with 5tbsp cooked brown, basmati rice.

● **Chicken tikka masala** Slice 1 medium, skinless, chicken breast fillet and simmer in 115ml/4floz Homepride 96% Fat Free Tikka Masala Sauce, until cooked through. Serve with 5tbsp cooked brown, basmati rice and a small green side salad. Plus 1 medium slice melon.

● **Mushroom omelette and chips** Whisk 2 eggs and mix with 1 handful sliced button mushrooms; 1tsp freshly-chopped herbs; and season to taste. Pour the mixture into a non-stick pan sprayed with one-cal spray oil. Cook thoroughly and serve with 100g pack McCain Microchips and 2tbsp peas.

● **Fish fingers and chips** Grill 4 fish fingers and serve with 150g/5oz cooked potatoes mashed with 2tsp low-fat spread and a little skimmed milk. Serve with 3tbsp green beans, sweetcorn or peas.

● **Veggie burger and chips** Grill 1 Quorn Quart Pounder and serve with 1 level tbsp Dijonnaise sauce, 100g pack McCain Microchips and 125g 4½oz frozen veggies.

● **Pasta bolognese** Brown 100g/3½oz extra-lean minced beef in a non-stick pan. Add 150ml/¼pt Dolmio Tomato And Chunky Mushroom Sauce and simmer for 20 minutes. Serve with 50g/2oz (dry weight) cooked pasta and salad.

● **Traditional chicken dinner** Serve 3 slices (100g/3½oz) skinned, lean, roast chicken with 100g/3½oz roasted potatoes; 1 medium portion of fresh green vegetables; carrots; and fat-skimmed gravy. Plus 1 satsuma or plum.

● **Chicken tortilla** Slice 1 small, skinless chicken breast fillet and stir-fry with 1 sliced red pepper in 1tsp olive oil and a little chilli sauce. When the chicken is almost cooked, add 1–2tbsp tomato sauce and finish cooking. Place in 1 Mexican tortilla wrap and serve with a green salad.

● **Veggie pasta** Cook 50g/2oz (dry weight) penne pasta, drain and stir into half a 400g can ready-made ratatouille. Sprinkle with 1 level tbsp grated Parmesan cheese and freshly-chopped basil.

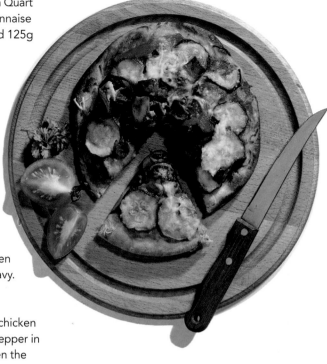

● **Pizza** Top 1 x 13cm/5in ready-made pizza base with 2tbsp Dolmio Tomato Pizza Sauce; vegetables of your choice; and 2 level tbsp grated reduced-fat mozzarella cheese. Bake in the oven until base is cooked through and the cheese is bubbling. Serve with a green side salad.

Snacks

APPROX 125 CALS

● 3 rich tea biscuits.
● 2 finger shortcake biscuits.
● 4 plain breadsticks with 1tbsp low-fat savoury dip.
● 25g/1oz Brie on 2 Ryvita Dark Rye.
● 2 cream crackers with 2 Laughing Cow Light Cheese Triangles and 1tsp sweet pickle.
● 100g/3½oz full-fat Greek yoghurt with 1tsp runny honey.

● 150g Müllerice 99% Fat Free.
● 1 individual choc ice.
● 1 Wall's Solero Citrus.
● 1 Cadbury Caramel Cake Bar.
● 1 chocolate mini roll.
● Any 125-calorie snack from the diets for apple

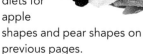

shapes and pear shapes on previous pages.

Snacks

APPROX 250 CALS

● 45g/1¾oz mixed nuts and raisins.
● 1 x 50g bar Cadbury Bournville chocolate.
● 1 standard-size Cadbury Dairy Milk chocolate bar.
● 1 x 34g pack crisps; 1 apple.
● Any 250-cal snack from the apple- or pear-shape diets on previous pages.

Don't forget to vary your meal choices so you get all the nutrients you need

EXERCISE

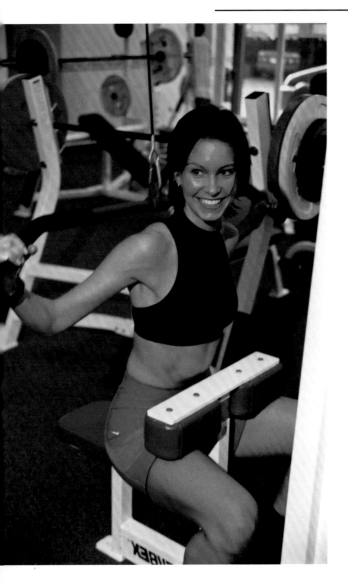

1 It makes your skin look great

Exercise doesn't only tone up what's under the skin, it will get you a cracking complexion, too. 'When we exercise we get warmer, which causes blood to flow to the skin's surface. This carries the oxygen and nutrients needed for a great complexion,' says fitness consultant Rachael Hill. So get busy with a workout and peachy skin could be yours for keeps.

2 You look slimmer instantly

Working out – especially programmes such as yoga or Pilates, which include exercises that concentrate on postural alignment, flexibility and muscle tone – is a great way to improve your posture and, as a result, you'll look immediately slimmer without counting so much as a single calorie. 'Someone who's 12st with good posture and strong abdominal muscles will look slimmer than someone who's a stone lighter but slouches,' says physiotherapist Robert Wood. Why do you think modelling schools spend so much time working on deportment?

3 You burn loads more calories – and not only when you're working out

It's common knowledge that if you exercise, you'll burn calories – but did you know that you'll carry on burning more calories after you stop? 'Yes, your calorie burning capacity stays elevated after you stop exercising,' says fitness consultant Rachael Hill. 'Because you increase your amount of lean muscle with exercise, particularly strength training, and muscle tissue requires more energy from the body than fat, your resting metabolic rate is higher. This means you'll not only burn extra calories when you're exercising but even when you're resting.' The thought that you'll be using up more calories just to watch Coronation Street should be more than enough impetus to get you into those jogging pants.

4 It boosts your mental powers

It has been scientifically proven that exercise can bring about a significant increase in brain power, improving memory and even offsetting possible mental decline due to age. A study carried out by the Duke University Medical Centre in North Carolina, America, showed that half an hour of physical exercise three times a week is enough to reap these benefits, which are believed to be down to the increased flow of oxygen-rich blood to the brain.

5 It works wonders on your flabby bits

It is possible to lose weight without exercising, but dieting alone ain't going to get you that six-pack. To get a toned tummy – or arms, or legs, or bum, for that matter – you need to adopt a regular fitness routine and, in particular, do

10 great reasons
to fall in love with exercise

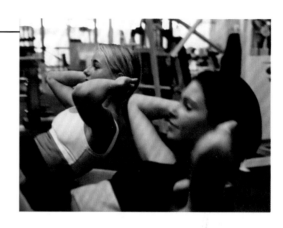

resistance training. Get yourself down the gym, buy a set of dumbbells from your local sports shop, or invest in a resistance band. It won't be long before you start toning up those long-despised flabby bits (and don't worry, doing weights won't have you mistaken for Popeye any time soon).

6 It beats stress and helps you sleep better

If you spend long nights tossing and turning and feel decidedly unrefreshed of a morning, working out could help. A recent study at Stanford University in the US showed that volunteers suffering from stress-induced sleep problems who did low-impact aerobics four times a week fell asleep more quickly, slept an hour longer than average and had a better quality sleep.

7 It gives you the 'feel good factor'

Exercising encourages the release of the hormone serotonin, which makes you feel good about yourself, and lifts the blues. 'People talk about the "runner's high" and anyone who doesn't exercise can't understand what that means,' says Dean Hodgkin, health and fitness consultant at Ragdale Hall Health Hydro. 'But it is a fact that exercise encourages the production of the body's natural opiates, causing definite improvements in mood.' And it's not only high-impact exercising like running that causes this effect – even a brisk walk will have you feeling happier.

8 It improves your sex life

Although bedroom antics are undoubtedly a form of exercise in their own right (burning around seven calories a minute so long as you don't just lie back and think of England), a regular exercise routine of the more orthodox variety will give your sex life a boost. 'Exercise increases flexibility, which can benefit your sex life because of the range of positions you'll be able to manage,' says fitness consultant Rachael Hill. 'And it develops muscle endurance, which will give you more sexual stamina.' In addition, because of the chemical rush of endorphins produced by physical activity, your sex drive could benefit from increased levels of DHEA, a hormone that boosts sexual excitement. On top of all that, working out helps beat fatigue, so you'll be less likely to feel too lacklustre for a roll in the hay come bedtime.

9 It keeps your bones in good order

Lack of exercise can lead to osteoporosis, the debilitating bone condition. Osteoporosis causes 60,000 hip and 50,000 wrist fractures each year, as well as loss of height and severe back pain. Currently one in three women and one in 12 men develop it, and, according to the National Osteoporosis Society, this figure is on the increase. A sedentary lifestyle is the major culprit because, like muscles, bones suffer if they're not used enough. Regular weight-bearing exercise, like walking, jogging or aerobics for at least 20 minutes a day is key to stopping brittle bones in their tracks.

10 You're more likely to stick to your diet

Finally, just how good do you feel after a thorough exercise session? If you've really worked at it, chances are the answer to this question is 'very'. And the lift you get from this exceedingly virtuous feeling, combined with the realisation that, yes, your arms are getting firmer or your waistband is becoming looser, means you're probably less likely to scoff a four-cheese pizza and a tub of ice cream when you get home after exercise. Working out will keep your mind focused on the job in hand and you'll be happy to go home and have lots of veggies with your meal instead of filling up on cheese slices. That way you'll feel even more smug the next time you step on those scales…

Your total body workout

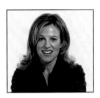

Fitness consultant Rachael Hill has devised three effective, fast and fun exercise programmes that will definitely work for you

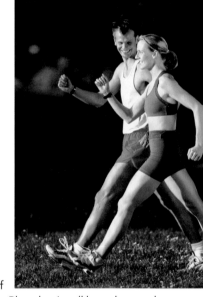

If you're not sure how long or hard you should be working out to lose weight, fitness consultant Rachael Hill has devised three new step-by-step programmes based on the simplest form of exercise there is – walking. All three routines are designed to blast calories and zap fat, and they include strength moves – so you'll be toning up those flabby bits at the same time.

Interested in a workout that's incredibly effective at toning muscles and burning off fat, that can be done in as little as 20 minutes, that doesn't involve membership fees, fancy workout gear or equipment, that will fit into any lifestyle and is so enjoyable that the time spent doing it disappears in an instant? Read on.

The workouts

For effective weight loss you should aim to do a minimum of 150 minutes of aerobic exercise a week. This may sound a lot, but you'll be amazed how quickly you can reach this target by slotting in a combination of the following 20, 30 and 40-minute workouts into your life.

Our three programmes include aerobic and resistance exercises designed to give you a total body workout and trim off inches. The activities in the workouts change every two or three minutes, so you'll never find yourself bored again. Plus, they're all based around walking so they can be done inside or outdoors, whenever it suits you. Now you really can use exercise to help you shed pounds and slim down – no matter how busy you are.

PHOTOGRAPHY: DAVID SMITH/ANDREW SYDENHAM/TELEGRAPH COLOUR LIBRARY. WITH THANKS TO TARA ALI.

5 STEPS to the perfect walking technique

If you want to turn walking into a fitness activity, observe these basic rules to avoid injury and burn maximum calories.

1 STAND TALL: Keep your chin up, back straight, stomach pulled in and shoulders back.

2 LIFT YOUR TOES: For a natural walking technique, your heel should strike the floor first then your foot should roll through to the toes. As you step, pull your toes up towards your shin. This may make your shins ache a bit at first but persevere. Your muscles will soon adapt and the ache will disappear.

How hard should I work?

LEVEL	PACE	APPROX SPEED	MINUTES PER MILE	HOW IT SHOULD FEEL
1	Easy	3mph	20	Admiring the view, leisurely stroll
2	Moderate	3.5mph	17	Going somewhere specific, purposeful walk to the shops
3	Brisk	4mph	15	Late for an appointment, breathing noticeably faster
4	Fast	4.5mph plus	13	On a mission, you can still hold a 'breathy 'conversation but probably prefer not to

The 20-minute workout

This workout is great if you want to fit in a quick exercise session before you leave for work or while the kids are occupied.

PERFECT FOR: toning, shaping and slimming your legs, thighs and bottom

CALORIES BURNED: 175 *

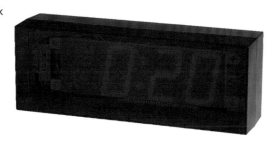

MINUTES 1 TO 4: WARM-UP
Start walking at level 1 and gradually increase to level 2. Concentrate on perfecting your technique.

MINUTE 5: STEP-OUT SQUATS
Stand with your hands on your hips. Facing forward, take a wide step out to the side with your right foot and slowly lower into a squat. Push your bottom backwards as though you're about to sit on a small stool and make sure your knees don't protrude forward past your toes. If it helps to balance, reach your arms out in front of you. Lower to the count of two and then, keeping your weight in your heels, push back up to the starting point. Repeat immediately on the left side.

NB This should be a continuous, flowing movement, squatting from side to side. You'll feel the muscles in the front of your thighs and your bottom working.

MINUTES 6 TO 8
Resume level 3 walking. Keep your arms pumping, your head up, stomach pulled in and your back straight.

MINUTE 9: WALKING LUNGES
Place your hands on your hips and take a large step forward with your right leg, slowly lunging until your right knee is at 90°,

taking care not to let the knee protrude past your toes. Hold for two counts. Then, pushing off on your right foot, bring the left foot forward to meet the right. Now step the left foot forward into a lunge, repeating the action.

MINUTES 10 TO 12
Resume level 3 walking.

Walking lunges

MINUTE 13: STEP-OUT SQUATS
As before.

MINUTES 14 TO 18
Resume level 3 walking.

MINUTES 19 TO 20: COOL-DOWN
Gradually decrease your walking pace until your breathing returns to normal.
Stretch thoroughly for five to 10 minutes.

*Approximate calorie values based on an 11st woman. The heavier you are, the more calories you'll burn.

3 AVOID OVER-STRIDING: The temptation to take longer strides increases as you walk faster but this can increase the risk of injury. Instead, try to take more frequent steps to increase your speed.

4 LEAN FORWARD: Imagine you are one long pole from your ankles to the top of your head. As you walk, try to lean forward slightly so that you feel you're almost falling forward into every step. Remember, the forward lean should come from your ankles, not from your waist, so that the rest of your body remains in a straight line.

5 USE YOUR ARMS: Bend your elbows slightly and then keep them in that position with your arms tucked into your sides. All the movement in the arms should come from a pendulum action at the shoulders, so they move like pistons and provide momentum. Avoid swinging your arms across the front of your body, though, as this is an inefficient use of your energy.

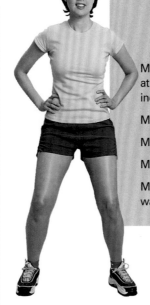

The 20-minute workout summary
For quick reference during your workout, copy this list to take with you.

Minutes 1 to 4: Start walking at level 1 and gradually increase to level 2.

Minute 5: Step-out squats.

Minutes 6 to 8: Level 3 walk.

Minute 9: Walking lunges.

Minutes 10 to 12: Level 3 walk.

Minute 13: Step-out squats.

Minutes 14 to 18: Level 3 walk.

Minutes 19 to 20: Decrease the pace until your breathing has returned to normal. Stretch thoroughly for five to 10 minutes.

Step-out squats

30-minute workout

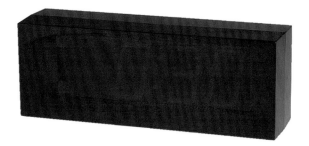

This workout is ideal if you don't have much time but still want to fit in an exercise session, eg in your lunch break. It works different parts of the body to the 20-minute workout so try to intersperse them.

PERFECT FOR: toning the arms and torso, as well as zapping loads of calories into the bargain
CALORIES BURNED: 225 *

MINUTES 1 TO 5: WARM-UP
Start walking at level 2 and build up to level 3. Focus on perfecting your technique.

MINUTE 6: TRICEP DIPS
Sit on the ground with your knees bent and your feet flat on the floor. Your palms should be flat on the floor behind you with your elbows tucked in and your fingers pointing towards your body. Slowly lower your body to the floor by bending your elbows behind you. Count to two as you lower and again as you lift. Repeat.
   To make this exercise harder, find either a park bench, a fixed bench in the gym or a heavy chair that won't tip. Sit on the edge with your legs straight and your feet out in front of you. Place your hands either side of your body and hold onto the edge of the bench seat, wrapping your fingers underneath it. Now lift your bottom off the bench, place your feet flat on the floor and bend your knees. Slowly lower your whole body towards the floor by bending at the elbows. Do this for a count of four

and then push yourself back up.

MINUTES 7 TO 10
Resume level 3 walk.

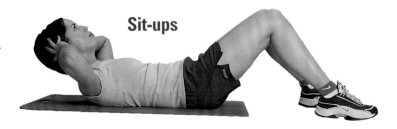
Sit-ups

MINUTE 11: SIT-UPS
Lie on the ground with your feet flat on the floor, knees bent and stomach pulled in throughout the movement. Place your hands at your temples. Slowly lift your head and shoulders off the floor to the count of two. Keep your head still and your chin lifted, then lower to the count of two. Repeat. Breathe out as you lift and in as you go down.

MINUTES 12 TO 14
Pick up the pace to a level 4 walk.

MINUTE 15: WAIST MINIMISER
Lie on the floor on your left side in a straight line. Support your upper body on the forearm of your left arm and bend both knees so that your feet are behind you and your knees are at 90°. Slowly raise your hips off the ground until you are in a straight line from your shoulders to your knees. Repeat. Lift to the count of four and lower to the count of four. Keep your stomach pulled in at all times and remember to breathe normally throughout.

MINUTES 16 TO 19
Resume level 4 walk.

MINUTE 20: WAIST MINIMISER
Repeat the above exercise on your right side.

MINUTES 21 TO 24
Resume level 3 walk.

MINUTE 25: BACK RAISES
Lie on the floor face down with your feet pointing out to the sides and your hands at your temples. Keep your forehead facing down to the floor and the back of your neck long. Slowly raise your chest off the floor until you can feel the muscles in your back beginning to work. Repeat. Count to two as you lift and then gently lower yourself back down again.

MINUTE 26
Resume level 3 walk.

MINUTES 27 TO 30: COOL-DOWN
Gradually decrease your walking pace until your breathing returns to its pre-exercise level. Stretch thoroughly for five to 10 minutes.

*Approximate calorie values based on an 11st woman.

Tricep dips

The 30-minute workout summary

For quick reference during your workout, copy this list to take with you.

Minutes 1 to 5: Start walking at level 2 and build up to level 3.

Minute 6: Tricep dips.

Minutes 7 to 10: Level 3 walk.

Minute 11: Sit-ups.

Minutes 12 to 14: Level 4 walk.

Minute 15: Waist minimiser, left side.

Minutes 16 to 19: Level 4 walk.

Minute 20: Waist minimiser, right side.

Minutes 21 to 24: Level 3 walk.

Minute 25: Back raises.

Minute 26: Level 3 walk.

Minutes 27 to 30: Decrease your walking pace until your breathing returns to its pre-exercise level. Stretch thoroughly for five to 10 minutes.

40-minute workout

This programme brings together exercises from both the shorter workouts for intensive, all-over fitness and toning. Try it at weekends or whenever you have a bit more time to enjoy it.

PERFECT FOR: conditioning the heart and lungs as well as the muscles, and increasing your fitness level in no time. This workout mixes short, calorie-busting intervals of fast walking with exercises from the 20 and 30-minute programmes for a workout that conditions your whole body.

CALORIES BURNED: 350 *

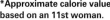

*Approximate calorie values based on an 11st woman.

MINUTES 1 TO 5: WARM-UP
Start walking at level 2 and gradually build up to level 3.

MINUTE 6: STANDING PRESS-UPS Stand approximately 2ft away from a wall. Place your hands on the wall at chest height, about one and a half times shoulder width apart. Slowly bend your elbows, keeping your body straight, until your nose is a couple of inches from the wall then gently push back to the starting position. Repeat.

MINUTES 7 TO 9
Resume level 3 walk.

MINUTE 10
Pick up the pace to a level 4 walk.

MINUTE 11: WALKING LUNGES
Place your hands on your hips and take a large step forward with your right leg until the knee is at 90°, making sure the knee doesn't protrude past the toes. Hold for two counts. Then, pushing off on your right foot, bring the left foot forward to meet the right. Now step the left foot forward into a lunge, repeating the action above.

MINUTES 12 TO 14
Resume level 3 walk.

MINUTE 15
Pick up the pace to a level 4 walk.

MINUTE 16: STEP-OUT SQUATS
Stand with your hands on your hips. Facing forward, take a wide step out to the side with your right foot and slowly lower into a squat. Push your bottom backwards as though you're about to sit on a small stool and don't let your knees protrude forward past your toes. If it helps to balance, reach your arms out in front of you. Lower to the count of two and then, keeping your weight in your heels, push back up to the starting point. Repeat immediately on the left. This should be a continuous movement from side to side. You'll feel the muscles in the front of your thighs and bottom working.

MINUTES 17 TO 19
Resume level 3 walk.

MINUTE 20
Turn up the heat by running on the spot as fast as you can.

Running on the spot

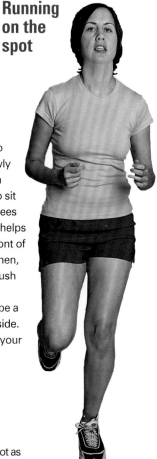

40-minute workout (continued)

Waist minimiser

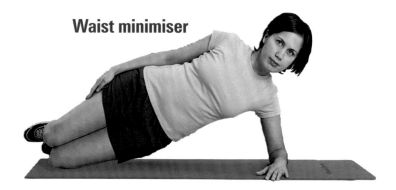

Stretch it out

It's important to stretch your major muscle groups thoroughly at the end of a workout, to avoid injury, release tension and to keep them long and sleek. Hold each stretch for 20 to 30 seconds on each side.

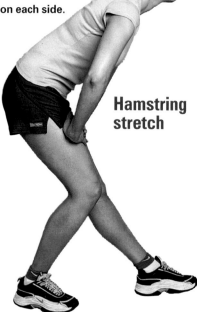

Hamstring stretch

MINUTE 21: BACK RAISES
Lie on the floor face down with your hands at your temples. Keep your forehead facing down and the back of your neck long. Slowly raise the chest off the floor until you feel the muscles in your back working. Count to two as you lift and then gently lower back down again for a count of two. Repeat.

MINUTES 22 TO 24
Resume level 3 walk.

MINUTES 25
Pick up the pace to a level 4 walk.

MINUTE 26: WAIST MINIMISER
Lie on the floor on your left side in a straight line. Support yourself on the forearm of your left arm and bend both knees so that your feet are behind you and your knees are at 90°. Slowly raise your hips off the ground until you are in a straight line from your shoulders to your knees. Repeat. Lift to the count of four and lower to the count of four. Keep your stomach pulled in at all times and remember to breathe normally.

MINUTES 27 TO 29
Resume level 3 walk. Remember to pull up your toes and strike the floor with your heel first.

MINUTE 30
Pick up the pace to a level 4 walk.

MINUTE 31: WAIST MINIMISER
Repeat on the right side.

MINUTES 32 TO 34
Resume level 3 walk.

MINUTE 35
Increase the pace to a level 4 walk.

MINUTES 36 TO 40: COOL-DOWN
Gradually decrease your walking pace until your breathing returns to its pre-exercise level. Stretch thoroughly for five to 10 minutes.

The 40-minute workout summary
For quick reference during your workout, copy this list to take with you.

Minutes 1 to 5: Start walking at level 2 and build up to level 3.

Minute 6: Standing press-ups.

Minutes 7 to 9: Level 3 walk.

Minute 10: Level 4 walk.

Minute 11: Walking lunges.

Minutes 12 to 14: Level 3 walk.

Minute 15: Level 4 walk.

Minute 16: Step-out squats.

Minutes 17 to 19: Level 3 walk.

Minute 20: Run on the spot.

Minute 21: Back raises.

Minutes 22 to 24: Level 3 walk.

Minute 25 : Level 4 walk.

Minute 26: Waist minimiser, left side.

Minutes 27 to 29: Level 3 walk.

Minute 30: Level 4 walk.

Minute 31: Waist minimiser, right side.

Minutes 32 to 34: Level 3 walk.

Minute 35: Level 4 walk.

Minutes 36 to 40: Decrease your walking pace until your breathing returns to its pre-exercise level. Stretch thoroughly for five to 10 minutes.

1 HAMSTRINGS (THE BACK OF THE LEGS)
Stand straight with your feet together. Step your left foot forward in front of you, then bend your right knee and sit into your right leg while keeping your left leg straight. Your knees should now be parallel. Place both hands on the top of your right leg to support your back. Keep your back straight and your chest lifted. Consciously stick out your bottom as you bend into the stretch. You should feel the stretch

from the back of the left knee up to the bottom. Breathe normally and hold that position for 20 to 30 seconds. As the tension wears off, try to ease a bit further into the stretch. Repeat on the other leg.

2 UPPER CALF MUSCLES AND UPPER BACK MUSCLE

Stand with your feet together and then take one large step back with your right foot. Make sure both your feet are pointing forward and that your back heel is directly behind your toes (don't let your back foot point away from your body). Keep your front knee bent and behind your toes, otherwise too much pressure will be placed on the knee joint. You should feel the stretch in the bulky part of your right calf muscle. As you do this, link your fingers together and push your arms out in front of you. Round your shoulders and feel the stretch across the upper back. Hold both stretches for 30 seconds before repeating on the other side. NB If you prefer, stand on the edge of a step or a curb or treadmill and drop your heel off the edge until you feel the stretch in your calf. If you want to stretch the lower part of the calf, too, simply bend your knee and sit into the stretch.

3 HIP FLEXOR, QUADRICEPS AND TRICEPS (THE FRONT OF THE HIP AND THIGHS AND THE BACK OF THE ARMS)

Kneel down on the floor and place your right foot in front of you with your knee bent. Slide your left knee backwards until you feel a stretch across the front of the thigh and the hip. Make sure that your right knee stays behind the toes of the right foot. Press your left hip forward into the stretch, then raise your right hand into the air and drop it behind your head. Use the left hand to create a stretch by gently pushing just below the elbow joint. You should feel a stretch between the armpit and the elbow of the right arm. Pull your stomach muscles in to avoid excessive arching of your

lower back. Hold the stretch for 20 to 30 seconds, breathing normally throughout. Repeat the stretch on the opposite side.

4 LOWER CALF, CHEST AND NECK Stand with your feet together and your back straight.

Move your right foot backwards slightly until your toes are just behind your left heel. Sit down into your back leg by bending both knees. You are trying to bring your shin closer to your right foot. You should feel a stretch around the lower calf. At the same time take your hands behind your back and grip your left wrist with your right hand. Gently lift the arms behind you while pushing your chest forwards. Feel the stretch across the front of your chest. Now drop your left ear to your left shoulder and stretch out one side of the neck. Hold all three stretches for 30 seconds before repeating them on the other side.

5 INNER THIGH AND SIDE STRETCH

Stand with your feet wide apart and turn your right foot out about 45°. Keep your hips facing forward and your back straight and bend into your right knee. Make sure the knee bends over the right foot but stays behind the line of the toes. The left foot should face forwards. Work the left foot away from the body until you feel a stretch along the inside of the leg. Hold that position while you place your right hand on your right thigh and reach up to the ceiling with your left arm.

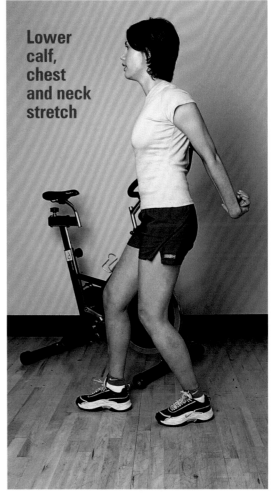

Lower calf, chest and neck stretch

Supporting the weight of your upper body on your right hand, gently push the left arm over the head, keeping it in line with the ear. You should feel a stretch down the side of the body. Hold both stretches for 20 to 30 seconds and then repeat on the other side.

Get fit facts

1 Contrary to popular thought, working out doesn't turn fat into muscle. You burn fat and tone muscle.

2 Resistance training won't create bulk, it'll give you toned muscle and help your body to burn energy quickly.

3 Stretching is the key to good flexibility and mobility in joints and muscles. This is very important as we age.

Your special occasion shape-up plan

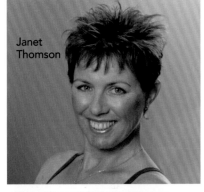

Janet Thomson

If you've got a special date to slim for, commit to being more active from today. Exercise is crucial – so fitness and nutrition expert Janet Thomson has created these three new plans. Stick with it and you can expect to drop a dress size in the first four weeks, and up to five sizes in a year!

How hard should I work?

When starting out on your plan, your heart rate and breathing will increase, and you'll start to feel warm. You will feel comfortable enough to say your name and address out loud, without becoming breathless. As you move into weeks two and three, you'll find it hard to chat during cardio sessions. By week four you'll feel hot and sweaty and your heart will pound. When toning, the final few reps should be a struggle but not painful. If they're too easy, do more reps, if you're struggling, stop when your muscles become painful.

TONING EXERCISES

These are the toning exercises you need to do as part of your personal four-week plan

ABDOMINAL CURL
Lie on the floor, knees bent. Pull in your transverse muscle (the corset-like muscle that wraps around your waist). Support your head, and curl forward. Don't pull on your neck as you curl up.

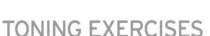

Abdominal curl

SQUAT
Stand with your feet apart and bend down, sticking your bum out until you sit back into your heels. Raise yourself back up, squeeze your buttocks and bring your weight onto the balls of your feet.

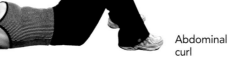

Box press-up

BOX PRESS-UP
On all fours, slide your knees behind your hips. Place your hands wider than your shoulders. As you lower your torso to the floor, pull your transverse muscle in, and keep your back flat.

LEG RAISE
Using a chair or wall for support, keep your hips square to the front and as you lift your leg, slightly tilt your pelvis forward and squeeze your buttocks.

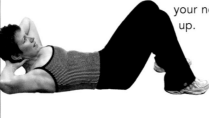

Leg raise

GOT 1ST TO LOSE? USE THIS PLAN

Your focus over the next four weeks will be on aerobic work, with some toning exercises,
to improve your fitness, so you can work harder and burn even more fat

WEEK 1	WEEK 2	WEEK 3	WEEK 4
Now's the time to start introducing your body to aerobic exercise. Learn how to use your tummy muscles by working the transverse muscles that wrap around your waist. They're vital for good posture and, if worked well, can trim inches off your waistline.	By now, you should have noticed your energy levels are a lot higher.	More of the same – with the emphasis on *more*!	This week, try and go for a real cardio boost!

WEEK 1

CARDIO
- *WALK/CYCLE*
5-7 mins every other day.

TONING
- *TRANSVERSE EXERCISE*
One set of 20 reps daily.
- *ABDOMINAL CURLS*
Starting on day four, 10 reps daily.

WEEK 2

CARDIO
- *WALK/CYCLE*
15 minutes at least five times this week. Walk harder with a longer pace and use your upper body more. If you're cycling, find a route with more hills that will challenge you.

TONING
- *TRANSVERSE EXERCISE*
One set of 20 reps daily.
- *ABDOMINAL CURL*
One set of 10 reps daily.
- *UPPER BACK*
One set of 15 reps (on the days you walk/cycle) at least five times this week.

WEEK 3

CARDIO
- *WALK/CYCLE*
25 minutes at least five times this week. Walk at the same pace as last week, but find a route that's challenging yet still comfortable.

TONING
- *TRANSVERSE EXERCISE*
One set of 20 reps daily.
- *ABDOMINAL CURL*
One set of 20 reps daily.
- *BOX PRESS-UP*
Start with one set of 10 repetitions daily and work up to one set of 15-20 repetitions by the end of this week.

WEEK 4

CARDIO
- *WALK/CYCLE*
Every day, do your 25-minute route 30 seconds faster. By the end of this week, you'll be covering your route 3$\frac{1}{2}$ minutes faster.

TONING
- *TRANSVERSE EXERCISE*
One set of 20 reps daily.
- *ABDOMINAL CURL*
One set of 20-25 reps four days a week.
- *BOX PRESS-UP*
One set of 20-25 reps four days a week.

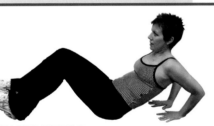

Tricep press

TRICEP PRESS
Sitting on the floor, place your hands slightly behind you, shoulder-width apart and your fingers forward. Bend your arms and lean back. To return to sitting, slowly extend your arms. Use your transverse muscle to keep your torso upright.

TRANSVERSE EXERCISE
Lie flat on your back, knees bent. Imagine your tummy muscles are like a belt around your waist with the buckle as your belly button. Do the belt up tighter and pull the buckle in tight – hold for six seconds, release. Do this 20 times a day. Check your plan for the number of reps you should do.

OUTER THIGH (TOP LEG)
Lie on your side and support your head in your hand – your top leg straight and in line with your hips and shoulders, your bottom leg bent. As you raise your leg slightly, rotate your foot forward towards the floor.

Outer thigh

INNER THIGH (BOTTOM LEG)
Lie on your side and bend your top knee in front and rest it on a pillow to keep your hips from rolling forward. Raise and lower your underneath leg.

OBLIQUE (WAIST)
Start as you would an abdominal curl – using your transverse muscle, but as you lift, rotate your torso so your shoulder, not elbow, goes towards your opposite knee.

Oblique

UPPER BACK
Stand with one foot in front of the other and lean onto your front leg so your torso is in a diagonal line with your back leg. Reach both arms forward, with a weight in each hand, and pull both elbows back and squeeze your shoulders together.

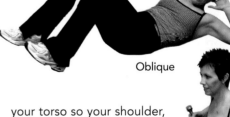

Upper back

GOT 2ST TO LOSE? USE THIS PLAN

Your focus over the next four weeks is toning. The only place in your body that burns fat is your muscles, so it's important to get them moving as much as possible

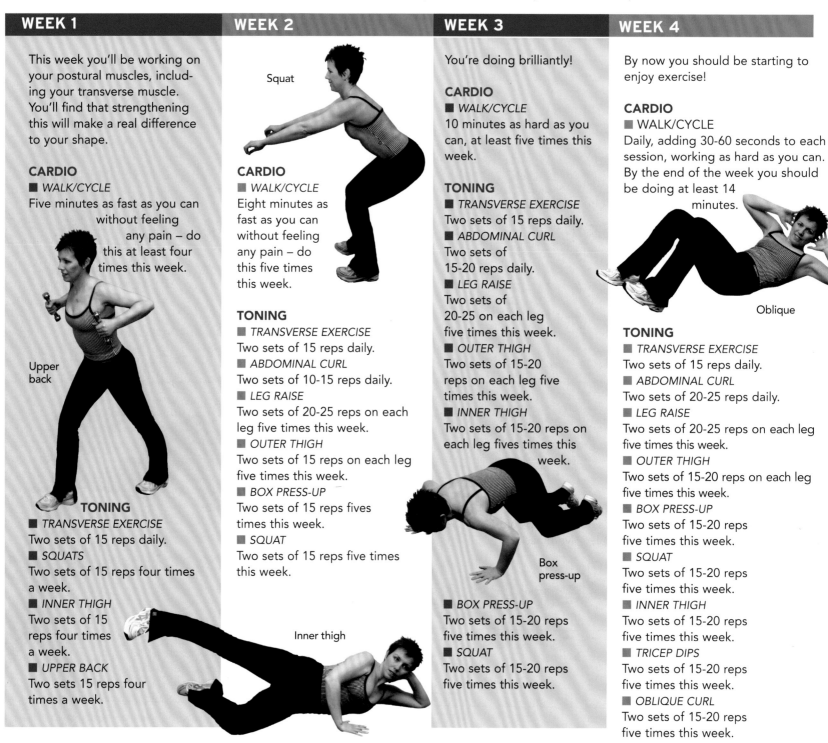

WEEK 1

This week you'll be working on your postural muscles, including your transverse muscle. You'll find that strengthening this will make a real difference to your shape.

CARDIO

■ *WALK/CYCLE*
Five minutes as fast as you can without feeling any pain – do this at least four times this week.

Upper back

TONING

■ *TRANSVERSE EXERCISE*
Two sets of 15 reps daily.
■ *SQUATS*
Two sets of 15 reps four times a week.
■ *INNER THIGH*
Two sets of 15 reps four times a week.
■ *UPPER BACK*
Two sets 15 reps four times a week.

WEEK 2

Squat

CARDIO

■ *WALK/CYCLE*
Eight minutes as fast as you can without feeling any pain – do this five times this week.

TONING

■ *TRANSVERSE EXERCISE*
Two sets of 15 reps daily.
■ *ABDOMINAL CURL*
Two sets of 10-15 reps daily.
■ *LEG RAISE*
Two sets of 20-25 reps on each leg five times this week.
■ *OUTER THIGH*
Two sets of 15 reps on each leg five times this week.
■ *BOX PRESS-UP*
Two sets of 15 reps fives times this week.
■ *SQUAT*
Two sets of 15 reps five times this week.

Inner thigh

WEEK 3

You're doing brilliantly!

CARDIO

■ *WALK/CYCLE*
10 minutes as hard as you can, at least five times this week.

TONING

■ *TRANSVERSE EXERCISE*
Two sets of 15 reps daily.
■ *ABDOMINAL CURL*
Two sets of 15-20 reps daily.
■ *LEG RAISE*
Two sets of 20-25 on each leg five times this week.
■ *OUTER THIGH*
Two sets of 15-20 reps on each leg five times this week.
■ *INNER THIGH*
Two sets of 15-20 reps on each leg fives times this week.

Box press-up

■ *BOX PRESS-UP*
Two sets of 15-20 reps five times this week.
■ *SQUAT*
Two sets of 15-20 reps five times this week.

WEEK 4

By now you should be starting to enjoy exercise!

CARDIO

■ WALK/CYCLE
Daily, adding 30-60 seconds to each session, working as hard as you can. By the end of the week you should be doing at least 14 minutes.

Oblique

TONING

■ *TRANSVERSE EXERCISE*
Two sets of 15 reps daily.
■ *ABDOMINAL CURL*
Two sets of 20-25 reps daily.
■ *LEG RAISE*
Two sets of 20-25 reps on each leg five times this week.
■ *OUTER THIGH*
Two sets of 15-20 reps on each leg five times this week.
■ *BOX PRESS-UP*
Two sets of 15-20 reps five times this week.
■ *SQUAT*
Two sets of 15-20 reps five times this week.
■ *INNER THIGH*
Two sets of 15-20 reps five times this week.
■ *TRICEP DIPS*
Two sets of 15-20 reps five times this week.
■ *OBLIQUE CURL*
Two sets of 15-20 reps five times this week.

GOT 3ST TO LOSE? USE THIS PLAN

Your focus over the next four weeks is to do a mixture of toning and aerobic exercises,
sometimes together in one session

WEEK 1

This week you'll be concentrating on aerobics. You'll also start doing the transverse exercise, which is vital for good posture. Once you've perfected this, do it anywhere – in the kitchen, at work or wherever you want, in fact.

CARDIO
- *WALK/CYCLE*
For 14 minutes at least five times this week. Work at a moderate pace for the first 2-3 minutes, then go as fast as you can for 8-10 minutes, then do another two minutes at a slower pace.

TONING
- *TRANSVERSE EXERCISE*
One set of 20 reps daily.
- *ABDOMINAL CURL*
Add two sets of 10-15 reps on day three, for the rest of the week.

WEEK 2

Now add toning exercises to your aerobic work.

CARDIO
- Repeat week one.

Abdominal curl

TONING
- *TRANSVERSE EXERCISE*
One set of 20 reps daily.
- *ABDOMINAL CURL*
Two sets of 10-15 reps daily.
- *BOX PRESS-UP*
Two sets of 15 reps five times this week.
- *LEG RAISE*
Two sets of 25 reps five times this week.
- *UPPER BACK*
Two sets of 20 reps five times this week.
- *INNER THIGH*
Two sets of 25 reps on each leg five times this week.
- *OUTER THIGH*
Two sets of 25 reps on each leg fives times this week.

WEEK 3

Try interval training:

TONING
Start your routine with these toning exercises:
- *TRANSVERSE EXERCISE*
Two sets of 10-15 reps daily.
- *ABDOMINAL CURL*
Two sets of 10-15 reps daily.
- *SQUAT*
Two sets of 15-20 reps daily.
- *TRICEP PRESS*
Two sets of 15-20 reps daily.
- *LEG RAISE*
Two sets of 20-25 reps on each leg five times this week.
- *OUTER THIGH*
Two sets of 15-20 reps on each leg five times this week.
- *SQUAT*
Two sets of 15-20 reps five times this week.
- *INNER THIGH*
Two sets of 15-20 reps on each leg five times this week.

CARDIO
- *THEN walk/cycle for 14 minutes as in week 2, and when you get back, do these:*

TONING
- *INNER THIGH*
Two sets of 20-25 reps on each leg.
- *OUTER THIGH*
Two sets of 20-25 reps on each leg.
- *BOX PRESS-UP*
Two sets of 15 reps.

WEEK 4

We're extending the interval training programme this week to include two bursts of aerobics. This is a challenging workout, but will shift those lbs. Aim to do it five times this week for maximum results in the shortest time.

Upper back

CARDIO
- *WALK/CYCLE*
For 15 minutes then do the following:

TONING
- *LEG RAISE*
Two sets of 25 reps on each leg.
- *SQUAT*
Two sets of 20 reps.
- *UPPER BACK*
Two sets of 15-20 reps.

CARDIO
- *WALK/ CYCLE*
Another 10 minutes to take you home, then finish with these:

TONING
- *TRANSVERSE EXERCISE*
Two sets of 10-15 reps.
- *ABDOMINAL CURL*
Two sets of 15- 20 reps.
- *OBLIQUES*
Two sets of 15-20 reps.
- *INNER THIGH*
Two sets of 25 reps on each leg
- *OUTER THIGH*
Two sets of 25 reps on each leg.

The plan

How it works: The exercises are divided into three stages to make up the six-week plan: Stage 1 should be done in weeks 1 to 2; Stage 2 covers weeks 3 to 4; and Stage 3 is for weeks 5 to 6.

Frequency: Do this workout at least three times a week, but don't overdo it at first. Take a day off between each session, as this will give your muscles time to rest.

The workout: For each exercise, do three sets of 12 to 15 repetitions, unless otherwise stated. If an exercise is too hard, do the easier option from the previous stage. If an exercise is too easy – ie you can easily do more than 12 to 15 repetitions in one go – do a harder one from the next stage. Let your muscles rest between each set or do an exercise that works a different area of the body before going back to do the next set.

Cardio crunchers

This programme will help create a leaner, more toned body, but it won't burn fat. You also need to do half an hour of aerobic exercise five times a week for this. Try some of these ideas:
◆ Set your alarm 30 minutes early and stick on a fitness video. If you're easily bored rent new ones from the library.
◆ Cycle to work and back. You'll probably end up doing more than 30 minutes a day – plus you'll save on travel costs.
◆ Play rounders in the park with workmates or friends.
◆ Don trainers and walk off any tension in your lunch hour.
◆ Buy an exercise bike and vow never to watch *EastEnders* again without pedalling away.

Tone up your wobbly bits in six weeks with our easy exercises

STOMACH
■ For stronger and flatter stomach muscles

Stage 1

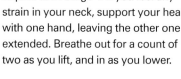

STAGE 1
ABDOMINAL CURLS
Lie on your back with your feet flat on the floor, knees bent and stomach pulled in. Place your hands at your temples. Slowly lift your head and shoulders off the floor to a count of two, then lower for a count of two. Keep your head still and your chin up. Breathe out as you lift up, and in as you lower.

STAGE 2
EXTENDED ARM ABDOMINAL CURLS
Lie down as in Stage 1. This time, extend your arms over your head.

Repeat as in Stage 1. If you feel any strain in your neck, support your head with one hand, leaving the other one extended. Breathe out for a count of two as you lift, and in as you lower.

STAGE 3
REVERSE ABDOMINAL CURLS
Lie down as in Stage 1, with your

hands at your temples. This time, raise your legs in the air. Slowly lift your head and shoulders off the floor for a count of two, and as you do so, raise your bottom a few inches off the floor, too. Don't rock your feet backwards and forwards, but lift them slightly as you raise your bottom. Breathe out as you lift, and in as you lower.

BACK
■ Works the muscles along the spine to create a straighter, taller, more flattering posture

STAGE 1
BACK RAISES
Lie on the floor, face down, with your

feet pointing outwards and your hands behind your back. Raise your chest off the floor until you feel a contraction in your back muscles. Breathe out and count to two as you lift, then lower down again for two counts, breathing in as you go.

STAGE 2
BACK RAISES WITH HANDS AT TEMPLES
Repeat as in Stage 1, but this time place your hands at your temples.

STAGE 3
EXTENDED BACK RAISES
Repeat as in Stage 1, but this time extend your arms over your head.

Stage 1

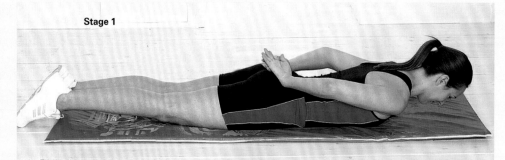

and TUMS

WAIST

■ Works on your tummy muscles for a defined waist and firmer stomach

STAGE 1
WAIST CRUNCHES

Lie on your back with your feet flat on the floor, your knees bent and your tummy pulled in. Place your hands at your temples. Slowly lift your head and shoulders off the floor to a count of two,

drawing your right shoulder across to your left knee. Lower to the count of two. After three sets, repeat on the other side.

STAGE 2
LYING HIP HITCHES

Lie on the floor on your left side, making sure the right leg is neatly stacked on top of the left. Wrap your left arm around your torso. Place your right hand on the floor in front of you at chest height. Lift your shoulders and right leg at the same time. Hitch

your right hip towards the right shoulder as you lift. As you do so, try not to put pressure on your right arm. Lift to a count of two and lower to a count of two. Breathe out as you lift, and in as you lower. After three sets, repeat on the other side.

STAGE 3
SIDE LYING HIP RAISES

Lie on the floor on your left side, with your body in a straight line. Support your upper body on your left forearm and bend both knees so that your lower legs are behind you and your knees are at 90°. With your forearm taking your body weight, slowly raise your hips off the ground until you're in a straight line from your shoulders to your knees. Lift to a count of four and lower to four. After three sets, repeat on the other side.

Stage 3

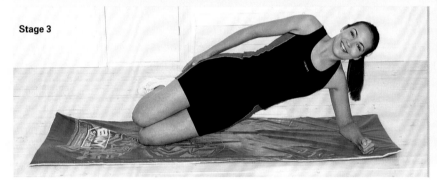

LEGS AND BOTTOM

■ For slimmer, leaner-looking legs

STAGE 1
SLIDING SIDE STEPS

Stand with your feet hip-width apart, with your bottom tucked in, and shoulders back and down. Take a large step sideways with your right foot, bending your knees as you go and lowering into a squat. Push your bottom backwards. As you push back up, drag your left foot in towards your right foot, pulling against the ground as you go to create resistance. Once you've returned to standing, repeat the movement, this time leading with the left leg. Do three sets of 20 to 25 repetitions.

STAGE 2
INNER THIGH LIFTS

Lie on your left side on the floor, with your left leg straight and in line with your torso. Place your right leg in front of you, so your right knee is in line with your hip. Rest your head on your arm, and place your right hand on the floor in front of your chest. Keep your toes pointing forward and lift your left leg toward the ceiling

as high as possible. Pause at the top position for a moment, then return to the starting position. After three sets, repeat on the other side.

STAGE 3
INNER THIGH TAPS

Lie on your left side with your legs straight, and stretch your left arm straight above your head. Rest your head on your outstretched arm. Bend your right arm so your palm is on the floor, in front of your chest. Raise your right leg a few inches and turn it outwards slightly from the hip, so your toes point up. Now start the movement by lifting your left leg up to your right leg until your heels touch, then lower your left leg. Keep your buttocks tight, and your hips at right angles to the floor. After three sets, repeat on the other side.

Stage 2

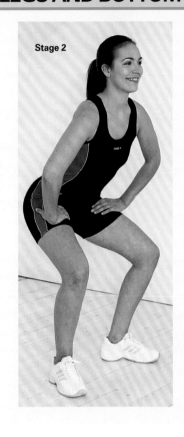

Stage 2

■ Targets all the muscles in the legs and bottom, helping to create a firm, toned, wobble-free bottom half

STAGE 1
SQUATS

Stand with your feet just over hip-width apart, with your toes angled outwards at about 45°. Slowly bend your legs, making sure that your knees stay in line with your toes. Try not to let your knees roll inwards. Lower yourself until your bottom is sticking out, a couple of inches above knee height. Your shoulders should be slightly past your knees, and your body weight should be over your heels, not your toes. Straighten your legs, pushing hard through your heels and keeping your body erect to return to the starting position. Lower to a count of two and lift to a count of two. Breathe normally throughout.

STAGE 2
WIDE SQUATS

Stand with your feet more than shoulder-width apart and your hands on your hips. Facing forward, take a wide step out to the right with your right foot, and slowly lower into a squat. Push your bottom backwards as though you're about to sit on a small stool, and make sure your knees don't protrude past your toes. If it helps you to balance, reach your arms out in front of you. Lower to the count of two and then, keeping your weight on your heels, push back up to the starting point for a count of two. Repeat straightaway on the left side. This should be a continuous, flowing movement, squatting from side to side. You'll really feel the muscles in your bottom and the front of your thighs working. You should also begin to feel warm and your breathing rate will increase.

STAGE 3
WEIGHTED SQUATS

■ The added weight works the muscles a little harder
Fill a well-fitting rucksack with three 2ltr bottles of water. Put it on your back, making sure it fits snugly to your body. Now do the exercise shown in Stage 1, making sure the rucksack isn't forcing you to lean forwards or backwards. Remember to push your bottom out but keep your shoulders above your knees throughout the exercise.

OUTER THIGHS
■ For strong outer thigh muscles

STAGE 1
BENT LEG OUTER THIGH RAISES

Lie on the floor on your side in a straight line, so that your shoulders and hips are at 90° to the floor. Support your head with your hand nearest the floor, and bend both knees by about 90° so that your lower legs are behind you. Slowly raise your top leg to a count of four, leading the movement with the knee and keeping the foot in line. Lower gently for a count of four. Remember to keep your hips at 90° to the floor at all times and don't let your hips drop backwards or forwards. Breathe normally throughout. After three sets, repeat on the other side.

Stage 1

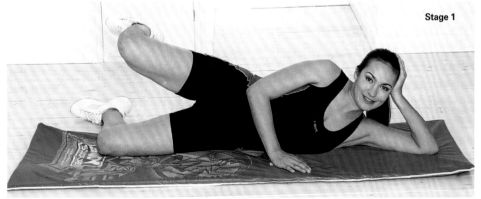

STAGE 2
STRAIGHT LEG OUTER THIGH RAISES

Repeat as in Stage 1, but this time straighten your top leg, keeping it in a straight line as you slowly lift and lower.

STAGE 3
TRAVELLING LEG OUTER THIGH RAISES

Repeat as in Stage 2, but this time slowly lift your leg to a count of two. Then, to a count of two, draw the knee across the body towards the chest, lowering it as you go, so that it almost touches the floor in front of you. Now straighten your leg to a count of two, leading the movement with your heel. Then slowly lower back to the starting position to a final count of two. Breathe normally throughout.

LEGS AND BOTTOM

■ Firms and strengthens your leg and buttock muscles

STAGE 1
STATIC LUNGES

Stand with your feet hip-width apart, your hands on your hips, your stomach pulled in, your shoulders back and your head held up. Take a large step forward with your right leg. From this position, slowly bend both knees and lower yourself down until your back knee is a couple of inches off the floor. At this point, check that there's a 90° gap at the back of both knees. Make sure your front knee doesn't protrude past your toes – keep it above your right heel and in line with your foot, so it doesn't roll in or outwards. Then use your legs to lift back up to the starting position. Lower to a count of four and lift to a count of four. Now change over so that your left foot is in front, and repeat the exercise. Breathe as normal throughout.

STAGE 2
ALTERNATING LUNGES

Stand with your feet hip-width apart, your hands by your sides, your stomach pulled in, your shoulders back and your head held up. In one smooth movement, take a large step forward with your right leg, lifting your arms in front of you to shoulder level. Lower down to a count of two, until your back knee is a couple of inches off the floor. At this point, both your knees should be bent at 90°. Check that your front knee does not protrude past your toes – keep it above your right heel and in line with your foot, so it doesn't roll in or outwards. Then use your legs to push yourself back up to the starting position, again to a count of two. Do three sets of 30 repetitions, alternating legs each time you step out. Breathe normally throughout. If you want to make this exercise harder, fill a well-fitting rucksack with three 2ltr bottles of water, placing it on your back before doing the move.

STAGE 3
TRAVELLING LUNGES

Place your hands on your hips, and take a large step forward with your right leg, lunging until your right knee is bent at 90°. Take care not to let your knee protrude past your toes. Hold for a count of two, then bring your left foot forward to meet your right. Now step your left foot forward into a lunge, repeating the action above. Do three sets of 30 repetitions, alternating your legs each time you step out. Breathe normally throughout. If you want to make this exercise harder, fill a well-fitting rucksack with three 2ltr bottles of water, placing it on your back before doing the move.

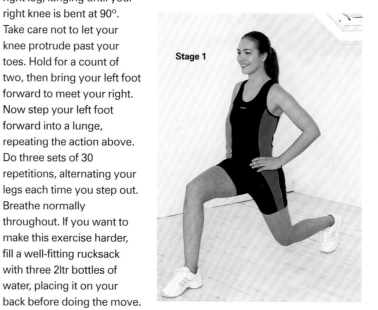

Stage 1

PROGRAMMES AT A GLANCE
Photocopy the following tick boxes to guide you though your workout and monitor your progress

STAGE 1

EXERCISE	SESSION 1	SESSION 2	SESSION 3	SESSION 4	SESSION 5	SESSION 6	SESSION 7
Ab curls (3 sets of 12 to 15 reps)	☐	☐	☐	☐	☐	☐	☐
Back raises (3 sets of 12 to 15 reps)	☐	☐	☐	☐	☐	☐	☐
Waist crunches (3 sets of 12 to 15 reps)	☐	☐	☐	☐	☐	☐	☐
Sliding side steps (3 sets of 20 to 25 reps)	☐	☐	☐	☐	☐	☐	☐
Squats (3 sets of 12 to 15 reps)	☐	☐	☐	☐	☐	☐	☐
Bent leg outer thigh raises (3 sets of 12 to 15 reps each side)	☐	☐	☐	☐	☐	☐	☐
Static lunges (3 sets of 12 to 15 reps each side)	☐	☐	☐	☐	☐	☐	☐

STAGE 2

EXERCISE	SESSION 1	SESSION 2	SESSION 3	SESSION 4	SESSION 5	SESSION 6	SESSION 7
Extended arm ab curls (3 sets of 12 to 15 reps)	☐	☐	☐	☐	☐	☐	☐
Back raises with hands at temples (3 sets of 12 to 15 reps)	☐	☐	☐	☐	☐	☐	☐
Lying hip hitches (3 sets of 12 to 15 reps)	☐	☐	☐	☐	☐	☐	☐
Inner thigh lifts (3 sets of 12 to 15 reps each side)	☐	☐	☐	☐	☐	☐	☐
Wide squats (3 sets of 12 to 15 reps)	☐	☐	☐	☐	☐	☐	☐
Straight leg outer thigh raises (3 sets of 12 to 15 reps each side)	☐	☐	☐	☐	☐	☐	☐
Alternating lunges (3 sets of 30 reps)	☐	☐	☐	☐	☐	☐	☐

STAGE 3

EXERCISE	SESSION 1	SESSION 2	SESSION 3	SESSION 4	SESSION 5	SESSION 6	SESSION 7
Reverse ab curls (3 sets of 12 to 15 reps)	☐	☐	☐	☐	☐	☐	☐
Extended back raises (3 sets of 12 to 15 reps)	☐	☐	☐	☐	☐	☐	☐
Side lying hip raises (3 sets of 12 to 15 each side)	☐	☐	☐	☐	☐	☐	☐
Inner thigh taps (3 sets of 12 to 15 reps each side)	☐	☐	☐	☐	☐	☐	☐
Weighted squats (3 sets of 12 to 15 reps)	☐	☐	☐	☐	☐	☐	☐
Travelling leg outer thigh raises (3 sets of 12 to 15 reps)	☐	☐	☐	☐	☐	☐	☐
Travelling lunges (3 sets of 30 reps)	☐	☐	☐	☐	☐	☐	☐

FEATURE: RACHAEL HILL. PHOTOGRAPHY: MARTIN SHAW

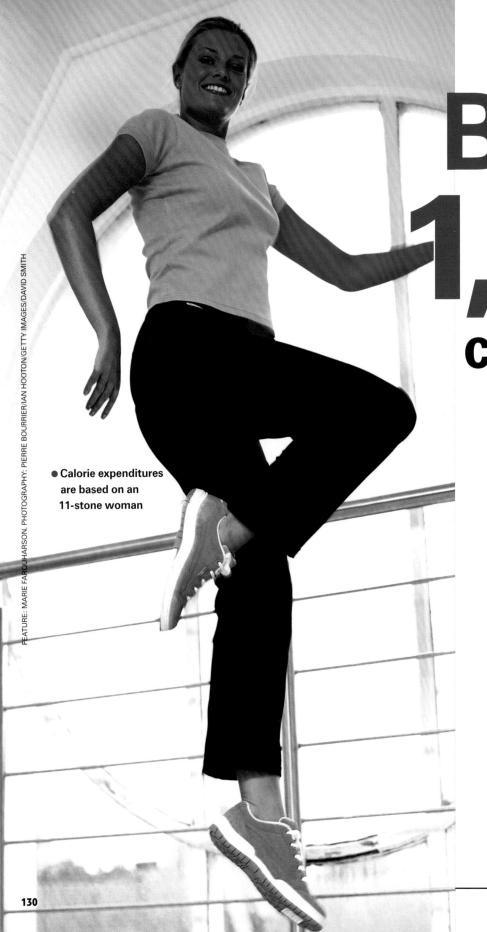

● Calorie expenditures
are based on an
11-stone woman

Burn *an extra* ∧
1,000
calories a day

Life's full of calorie-burning chances.
Here are five easy plans to zap 1,000…

Get up and go

79 calories Put on your favourite CD and
dance around the room for 15 minutes.

140 calories Walk up the stairs as many
times as possible each day. Just 15 minutes will
reap rewards.

246 calories At work, deliver messages to
colleagues in person rather than e-mailing. You
could tot up a couple of miles walking a day!

316 calories Partner up with a friend and go
to a 45-minute aerobic class after work or at
lunchtime.

240 calories Sort through your clothes for an
hour – and give away any you haven't worn for a
year.

TOTAL: 1,021 CALORIES

Enjoy the outdoors

70 calories Start your day with 10 minutes of t'ai chi. Not only will it help to tone you up, but it will also destress you and help you to focus on the day ahead.

180 calories Spend 30 minutes tidying up your garden, mowing the lawn and pulling up the weeds.

120 calories Spend 10 minutes skipping in your garden.

188 calories Go for a leisurely 15 minute after-dinner bicycle ride.

30 calories Play 10 minutes of croquet out in the back garden.

422 calories Take a hike into the country for a picnic. Allow yourself an hour for the round trip.

TOTAL: 1,010 CALORIES

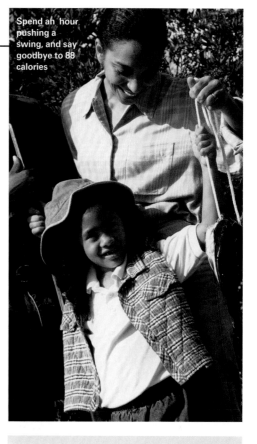

Spend an hour pushing a swing, and say goodbye to 88 calories

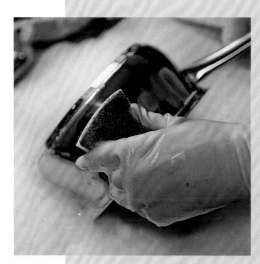

Want to burn 60 calories? Half an hour washing up will do the trick

Housework

246 calories Spring clean your kitchen and don't spare the elbow grease. After an hour, your body will have benefited as much as the floor.

167 calories Give your grubby windows a half-hour cleaning overhaul.

422 calories Spend an hour rearranging your bedroom furniture. According to the principals of feng shui, it'll boost your energy levels as well.

360 calories Spend an hour washing, waxing and vacuuming every inch of your car, from the hubcaps to the roof.

TOTAL: 1,195 CALORIES

Family time

140 calories Play an energetic game of catch or frisbee with the kids for 30 minutes.

360 calories Hit the ice rink with your family and do a Torvill and Dean for 40 minutes. Don't expect to impress the kids...

123 calories Walk the dog around the block for 30 minutes.

60 calories Paddle around a lake at a leisurely pace for 10 minutes.

156 calories Spend an hour cooking up one of your famous Sunday roasts with all the trimmings (low-calorie, low-fat versions of course!)

240 calories Hit the supermarket for your weekly family shop – it should take about an hour. Remember to write your shopping list before you go – that way you'll only come home with what you need, not lots of tempting extras.

TOTAL: 1,079 CALORIES

Spend an hour . . .

300 calories Massage out the knots in your partner's back and shoulders.

110 calories Turn off the computer and handwrite a letter to an old friend.

240 calories Sort out the clutter in the garage and decide what goes to charity.

360 calories Do a bit of decorating – give your spare room a lick of fresh paint.

TOTAL: 1,010 CALORIES

Swim

Regular visits to your local pool will kick your metabolism into high gear and get rid of pounds – fast

When you swim, every muscle is used to push against the water's resistance. It's great for your joints, it will tone and strengthen your muscles and it's also a fantastic all-round calorie burner. But if a trip to the pool is more likely to find you splashing around the shallow end than zooming up and down the fast lane, don't despair. We've put together some simple tips to ensure that the time you spend in the pool is 100% more effective.

How to burn more calories with each stroke

Once you've improved your swimming technique, you go faster, feel lighter, swim more efficiently and have more fun.

1 Start by standing in the shallow end of the pool and practising the breast stroke action with your arms – you may look a bit silly, but it'll be worth it! Keep your fingers together (gaps between them let the water rush through, reducing your ability to pull yourself forward). Cup your hands slightly and hold them in front of you at chest height with the back of your hands pressed together. Slowly push your hands forward, leading with your fingertips as you straighten your arms. Once your arms are almost fully extended, part your hands and begin to push back and down until your arms are

yourself SLIM

behind you. Now quickly pull your hands back to the starting position.

2 Try holding on to the side or use a kick board as you practise moving your legs. Pull your heels up to your bottom and then quickly push them out to the side as though drawing two large circles with your feet, before drawing your heels back up to your bottom again. Once you feel practised at doing the arms and the legs separately, try doing them both together.

3 Take care not to rush your strokes. It's better to perform a stroke well and feel the pressure on your pectoral muscles (the muscles across your chest) than to do lots of short, sharp movements that simply result in you feeling a bit uncomfortable and out of control.

4 Once you've swum up and down the pool a few times, try counting the number of strokes that you are doing per length (or width), then work on reducing this number. This will really help your overall technique because the fewer movements you use to cross the pool, the more efficient your stroke will become.

5 Starting off and turning around correctly at the end of each length will help to establish a continuous rhythm to your swimming pattern. To maximise your turns, keep your eyes fixed on the wall until you touch, then simply turn around and push off in as streamlined a position as possible. The less resistance you create, the further you will travel.

6 Once you feel confident in the pool try swimming faster for just one length and then take as many lengths as you need to get your breath back. As soon as you feel recovered, do it again. This will not only build up your stamina and increase your fitness levels but it will also mean you burn 20% more calories with each 'fast' length you do.

WHAT YOU GET

Water acts as a natural resistance to the body, which is why swimming is a great way to create a strong, toned, lean body.

CALORIES BURNED: Between 250 and 500 calories an hour. So, if you swim for a minimum of 30-45 minutes per day for three to five days of every week, you can expect to lose between 2lb-6lb of body weight in around six weeks.

HEALTH BENEFITS: Thirty minutes of swimming a day can lower your blood pressure, reduce your cholesterol, strengthen your heart and lungs and improve your circulation. If you haven't been active for a while, swimming is a very good way of easing yourself back into exercise and because water supports the entire body as it moves, it's ideal for anyone who is overweight or suffering from joint problems.

7 Improve your strokes by introducing simple 'drills'. For example, doing two breaststroke kicks to every one arm pull will strengthen your legs. Alternatively try catch-up freestyle – this means you finish one complete arm pull before starting the next. When you have mastered this, you can improve your stroke further by touching your hip, shoulder and head as you complete an arm pull, so ensuring your elbow remains in the correct place for a good freestyle stroke.

8 If you want to swim well, it's important to be comfortable with putting your face in the water. If you find this difficult, try wearing a pair of goggles to protect your eyes and practise breathing out as you put your head under water for a few short seconds at a time.

9 Choose a suit that's supportive, so you feel comfortable in the water. Online lingerie and swimwear retailer, Figleaves (www.figleaves.com), offers an extensive range of swimwear in larger cup sizes. We particularly love the Bioform swimsuit, which incorporates

technology from Charnos to flatter your shape and is available in sizes up to a 38-back and an F cup. Plus, shopping with an online retailer means you can choose from a wide range of swimwear all-year round.

10 It's important to drink plenty of fluids during and after swimming. As you're submerged it's easy to forget that the exercise is probably making you sweat – even though it isn't noticeable while you're in the water!

QUICK TIP

Rinse before and after you swim so chemicals don't dry out your skin. Protect your locks from chlorine damage by applying lots of conditioner under a latex swimming cap.

FEATURE: RACHAEL HILL. PHOTOGRAPHY: GETTY IMAGES

Fitness mistakes ruin your

Are you exercising regularly but not seeing the results you want? Check our guide to common fitness mistakes – it could make all the difference

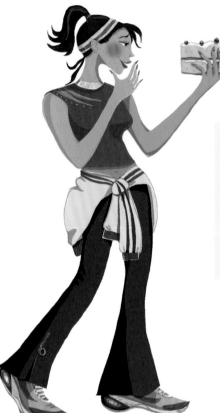

The mistake: Allowing yourself that extra cake after exercise

Contrary to popular belief, moderate exercise does not increase hunger levels. In fact, working out can slightly decrease the appetite. However, when faced with something particularly tempting it can be all too easy to convince yourself that it's OK to have a bit extra because, after all, you have exercised today. 'Don't do it,' says Penny Hunking, Director of Energise Nutrition. 'A piece of chocolate cake can be eaten in a flash but burning off the calories it contains will take more than an hour of solid exercise.'

The mistake: Not doing regular weight training

'People often focus on "aerobic" training when trying to lose weight,' says Matt Roberts, author of *Fitness for Life Manual.* 'However, resistance training (exercise that works the muscles using weights, exercise bands or machines) is crucial to weight loss.' This is because muscle needs a lot of calories to exist, so the more muscle you have the more calories you'll burn. 'Without regular weight training, adults will lose 5lb to 7lb of muscle tissue every decade,' says Anita Bean, author of *The Complete Guide to Strength Training.* 'This loss leads to a drop in the rate at which you burn calories.'

The mistake: Not warming up or cooling down

When you're pressed for time, it can be tempting to skip your warm-up or cool-down. Don't. A good warm-up gets your body ready to go and reduces the risk of injury. It boosts circulation, making muscles more pliable and ligaments more resilient, and helps joints move more easily. Loosen up your joints, then do five minutes of aerobic exercise, such as walking or cycling, until you feel warm.

A good cool-down allows the body to return to a pre-exercising state. Going from top gear to a sudden stop may cause you to feel dizzy, sick and faint, as blood pools in the legs. By slowing down gradually, blood is efficiently re-routed back to the major organs and the waste products that accumulate in your muscles during exercise are removed. Again, walk it out or cycle gently for five minutes until your breathing and heart rate come down. Then stretch out all your major muscles.

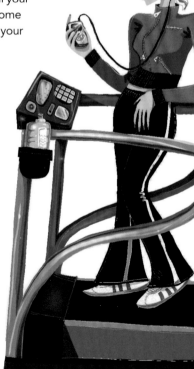

The mistake: Believing that gyms and leisure centres are for people who are already fit

'Gyms are in fact ideal places to go in order to improve fitness,' says Magnus Bowden, Group Gym Development Manager for Cannon Health Clubs. 'Talking to and exercising alongside like-minded people is great for support and motivation.' Gyms aren't

FEATURE: RACHAEL ANNE HILL. ILLUSTRATIONS: LUCY TRUMAN

that
workout

The mistake: Taking it too easy

If you don't work hard enough, changes to your body will be slow in coming, which could well demotivate you. During an aerobic session you should feel considerably warmer than normal and your breathing should increase to a point where you can still talk, but not without a little puffing and panting. When lifting weights or doing body conditioning exercises you shouldn't be able to do more than a maximum of 15 repetitions. Otherwise your muscles are not being sufficiently challenged.

The mistake: Working too hard

You don't have to exercise to a point where you're hot, sweaty and out of breath for it to do you good. 'Exercising at an intensity where you can hold a conversation will produce excellent health benefits and burn plenty of calories, too,' says fitness coach Bob Smith. 'It doesn't have to be hell to be healthy.' Although you should up the pace as you get fitter, you're working too hard if you get really hot, have difficulty breathing and generally feel very uncomfortable.

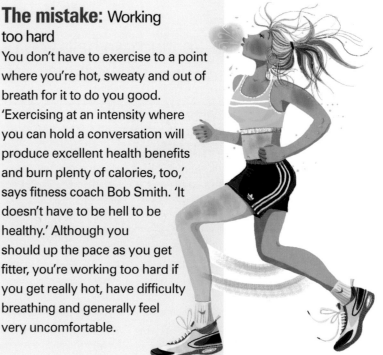

about skinny fanatics – just as many people like you are simply trying to tone up and slim down. And everyone – even a seasoned gym user – has to do an induction session in which trained staff show you how to use all the equipment and design you a personal fitness plan.

The mistake: Expecting results too quickly

'Exercise will not transform your body overnight,' says fitness consultant and athletics coach Bob Smith. 'It may have taken 10 years or longer to become the shape you are today so it stands to reason that your body can't completely change in a matter of a few short weeks.' Although you will notice bits toning up and slimming down in a few weeks, it can take several months to see a big difference in body shape. However, you'll notice many other benefits in the meantime, such as increased energy levels, reduced stress and a more positive outlook.

The mistake: Not setting clear exercise goals

'It is important to set goals with specific measures so that you can see how you are doing,' says Matt Roberts. 'Plan your workouts carefully, too. Not just for your next session but also for the coming four to six weeks.' For example, if you're doing two cardio workouts a week, plan to increase the amount you walk, jog or cycle etc by one or two minutes each session. If you've started on 10 minutes, after just four weeks you'll be able to keep going for at least 18 minutes.

The mistake: Sticking to the same old workout

Don't use the same fitness machines all the time or do the same aerobic workout week after week. 'Variety is key,' says Matt Roberts. 'The more you keep doing of the same thing, the less effective it becomes.' This is because your body gets used to the activity and no longer needs to

adapt to do it. Vary your exercises and keep pushing yourself as your fitness increases. Exercise for a few minutes longer every week, run, cycle or walk that bit faster, or lift slightly heavier weights. This way your body will keep adapting so that your level of fitness continually improves.

The mistake: Not drinking enough water

'If you don't drink enough water, you will tire more quickly during exercise,' says Anita Bean, who has also written *The Complete Guide to Sports Nutrition* 'You will probably need to drop the intensity (slow down or decrease the resistance) or stop early.' Exercise always feels harder if you are even slightly dehydrated because your heart and lungs have to work harder. It's only once you're dehydrated that you feel thirsty, so drink water early in your workout, before you feel thirsty. Aim to drink 1/2ltr for every 30 minutes you exercise – more in hot weather.

Eat to boost your fitness plan

It's true – eating can help you burn off calories more efficiently. Here's how

The food rules

- If you're working out regularly, the basic rule is that you'll need more fluids and carbohydrates to fuel the body.
- First, remember to drink water and plenty of it – aim for 2ltr a day. 'Always drink before, during and after your workout,' says sports dietician Jennette Higgs. 'Being properly hydrated will increase your energy, allowing you to work harder and burn more calories,' she says.
- Then, for optimal energy and performance, eat 200 to 300 calories an hour and half before you work out. Opt for carbohydrates like fat-free yoghurt and a banana or a cracker with peanut butter, including them in your allowance.
- And you'll need to replace lost energy stores after your workout. When you exercise you use glycogen – the body's stored form of carbohydrate – in your muscles for energy; and by the end of a session your muscles will be starved of glycogen. 'The best time to replace these reserves is in the first half hour to an hour after exercise when your body will best absorb it,' says Jennette. 'Eating a carb-rich meal after exercise helps replace lost energy, and so also helps you control your appetite.' What's more, if your body doesn't have enough carbohydrate it can't burn fat for fuel. Instead, it'll start breaking down muscle. With less muscle your metabolism will slow down and you'll burn less fat.
- So how do these rules fit in with your personal exercise schedule?

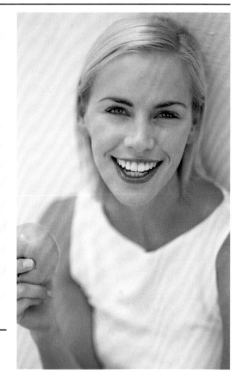

FEATURE: MARIE FARQUHARSON. PHOTOGRAPHY: MARIO SALAZAR

For the morning workout

If you don't have time for or can't stomach eating as soon as you wake up, don't head out for your exercise session without drinking a large glass of water first. 'Because you've had nothing to eat or drink overnight, your first priority is to hydrate yourself,' says Jennette. Start drinking before the session and sip throughout it. Straight after your session, you should rehydrate your body further. 'Commercial isotonic sports drinks are a good choice as they provide the right balance of sugars, salts and fluids lost through sweat', says Jennette. 'For a home-made version, try a very diluted orange juice and soda water: it's just as effective and much cheaper. For a quick shot of early morning energy, eat a handful of raw cereal or a small banana while you pull on your exercise gear.' If you've got a bit of time during your journey to the gym, eat a banana on the way or have half your normal breakfast bowl of cereal or a piece of wholemeal toast before leaving. Straight after your workout is when to eat a proper breakfast. If you're at home, have your normal bowl of cereal. If you go to the gym before work, a fruit bun and banana make an instant breakfast to stash in your bag. 'If you don't eat soon after your workout you'll feel so hungry you may end up bingeing,' says Jeanette.

For the lunchtime workout

If afternoon workouts fit better into your lifestyle, you need to eat some food an hour and a half before going to the gym. 'If you've had a sustaining breakfast you may need only a large glass of water before your session. If you know you'll need something more substantial, though, have a high-carb snack like a bagel and piece of fruit,' says Jennette. You could try to use part of your normal lunch, say, half of your sandwich, as a pre-exercise snack for your lunchtime or after-work workout.

For the evening workout

To avoid the end-of-day slump that might make you cry off the gym, have a snack at 4pm. 'If you're driving to the gym after work, eat fruit on the way,' says Jennette. 'If you need something more substantial, a scone and strawberries, dried fruits or a small bag of trail mix are good sources of easily digestible, instant energy, but save some calories from your allowance for this. Avoid high-fat foods before exercise as these sit heavily on the stomach.'

SUCCESS STORIES

How did Jane McDonald
shift the pounds?

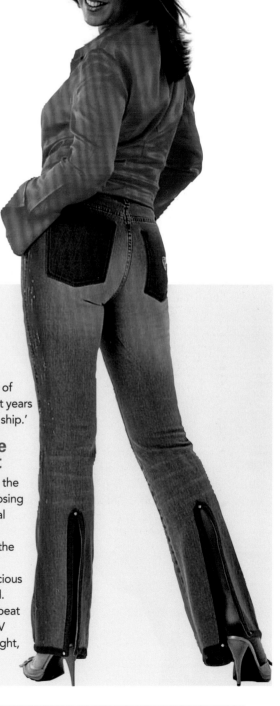

Jane McDonald talks to Lara Kilner about losing
1½st and gaining a new body and healthy glow

Docusoaps seem to have taken over TV in recent years and with them come characters for us to love or hate. One 'real-life' performer who's captured public affection is Jane McDonald, star of the BBC's The Cruise. Her strong voice and down-to-earth personality have made her a household name. Not only can she boast a number one album and a devoted fan base, she now has the looks to match her celeb status. Over the past year, Jane has embarked on a home exercise plan and cut down on cakes to drop four dress sizes. Here she gives us the new-look lowdown.

Jane on why the pounds piled on in the first place

'The excess weight crept on gradually when I was working on the cruise ship. It's a sociable lifestyle and most of it revolves around food. You eat so much, it's ridiculous – there's 24-hour service. I never did any exercise because I had to pass the cafeteria to actually get to the gym! I'd think, "Forget it" and sit down with a cup of tea and a pastry instead. A typical day for me would start with a big breakfast, then I'd meet someone for coffee and a slice of cake at around 11, then it'd be lunch, then afternoon tea, then dinner and then a midnight buffet – that's a lot of food over the eight years I was on the cruise ship.'

On why she lost weight

'I was content with the rest of my life, so losing weight was the final thing to do. Plus, suddenly being in the limelight meant I became very conscious of the way I looked.

'There was a repeat of The Cruise on TV recently and I thought,

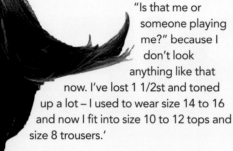

'My main secret is that I eat the same things I always have, but now I halve the portions – apparently Cindy Crawford does the same thing!'

"Is that me or someone playing me?" because I don't look anything like that now. I've lost 1 1/2st and toned up a lot – I used to wear size 14 to 16 and now I fit into size 10 to 12 tops and size 8 trousers.'

On discovering exercise

'I've got really into exercise and it's changing my shape. I feel far healthier now and the good thing is that when you're working out, you're not thinking about food. I'm too busy to go to the gym on a regular basis so I work out at home in the evenings, just before I go to bed. It helps me sleep better and it's nice to know that I don't have to get up and exercise – I hate mornings.

'I do toning work for 15 minutes every day – not excessive, but enough to make a difference. I use dumbbells and do two sets of 12 repetitions of each exercise. My main priority is my upper body. I'm lucky in that I have small legs and hips, but I'm top heavy. I have big boobs and am working on my arms – I've just about got rid of my 'wings' [the flabby bits under the upper arms].

'I've taken up Pilates, too. I went to a class to learn all the postures and then I practised at home. I do 15 minutes a day and feel so much better for it. My posture has improved, which makes me look slimmer.

'The other thing is that I only ever used to walk as far as my car but now I take a lot of brisk walks. It's a great way to improve your fitness without feeling like you're doing formal exercise.

'My job does help – I have a big projection in my voice and you use your abdominal muscles when you sing like that, so I've a well-toned tummy. Nerves are the other thing – I get very nervous before a show, which means I don't eat much. I'm sure the adrenalin rush must help burn calories, too!'

On curbing the cakes

'I eat a lot of salads and low-fat sandwiches, and I've found that I actually like them more than I used to. My tastebuds have changed – I used to eat loads of cake but now it tastes too rich.

'My main secret, though, is that I eat the same things I always have, but I halve the portions – apparently Cindy Crawford does the same thing, so there must be something in it! I don't deprive myself of anything, although I keep a check on my fat intake – one of my big weaknesses is crisps, so I'll have Jacobs Thai Bites (which are baked and rice- based so they're low in fat) instead, and I'll only buy a small bag. I don't have things in the house that I'm cutting down on, either – there might be a big bowl of fruit on the table, but if I know there's a Crunchie in the fridge, I'll want it. If it's not there, I can't eat it, can I?

'I never go hungry – the trick is to eat slowly, that way your brain tells you when you're full and you don't just keep on eating. Talking a lot helps too – something I'm good at! I put down my knife and fork after every mouthful and always try to carry on a conversation.'

On how great life is now

'I've got much more inner confidence and I'm sure that has a positive effect on my performance. I feel sexy, I have a glow and I know I look good in my stage outfits. I love the fact that I can look trendy, too. I always dressed in very floaty things before – I wouldn't wear anything tight because I had all these rolls of fat.I looked older than I was, too – although the perm didn't help. I will never have that hairstyle again! But now, I know I look good, and it's a great feeling that affects every area of my life.'

Jane's top diet tips

Don't feel guilty if you have a binge occasionally – if you want to finish off a bottle of wine or eat a bag of crisps, do so and enjoy it, but make sure you get yourself back on track the next day – just because you've fallen off the wagon doesn't mean you have to give up your healthy eating plan altogether.

Get a friend to motivate you – my backing singer, Sue, is really healthy and helps to keep my eating in check. We have caterers on tour and whenever I reach for the pudding, she'll say 'Jane, you don't really need that, do you?' which more often than not makes me put it back.

If you're craving something, it's OK to give in to it – in moderation. If I'm hankering after chocolate, I'll have a couple of chocolates rather than the whole box – that way it'll satisfy my craving and I won't need any more. It's all about re-educating your relationship with food.

Only eat when you're hungry – never just for the sake of it.

Keep a rein on your portion sizes – if you're enjoying something, it's so easy to keep on eating but I've learned to keep that in check. Just put less food on your plate and don't have things you're trying not to eat in the house, then you won't succumb to temptation.

Drink as much water as you can possibly manage – to flush out the toxins and fill you up. Have a bottle of water with you wherever you go.

Eat slowly – if you make food last longer, your stomach tells your brain that it's full, so you're less likely to overeat.

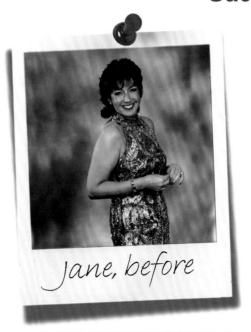

Jane, before

'Put less food on your plate and don't have things you're trying not to eat in the house, then you won't succumb to temptation'

Get Jane's arms

Invest in a set of dumbbells consisting of different weights so that you can increase the weight as your strength improves. Then, tone up your arms like Jane McDonald with these exercises. Do two sets of 12 repetitions at least every other day.

Tricep dips

To work the back of your arms, sit on the ground with your knees bent and your feet on the floor. Your palms should be flat on the floor behind you with your elbows tucked in and your fingers pointing towards your body. Slowly lower your body towards the floor to a count of four by bending your elbows behind you before returning to the original position.

Chest press

This tones your arms by working the back of your arms as well as your chest muscles. Lie on your back on the floor (or on a workout bench) and, holding a weight in each hand, bend your arms out to the sides with your elbows at 90° and the weights held up towards the ceiling. Push upwards to a count of four until your arms are nearly straight. Return to the starting position.

Bicep curl

This gives great tone to the upper arms. Stand with feet hip-width apart, knees slightly bent, and arms by your sides. Start with your elbows slightly bent, holding the weights a little in front of you with your palms facing forwards. Bend your elbows and lift the weights up towards your shoulders to a count of four before lowering. Keep the elbows tucked in close to your body. The movement should be slow and smooth.

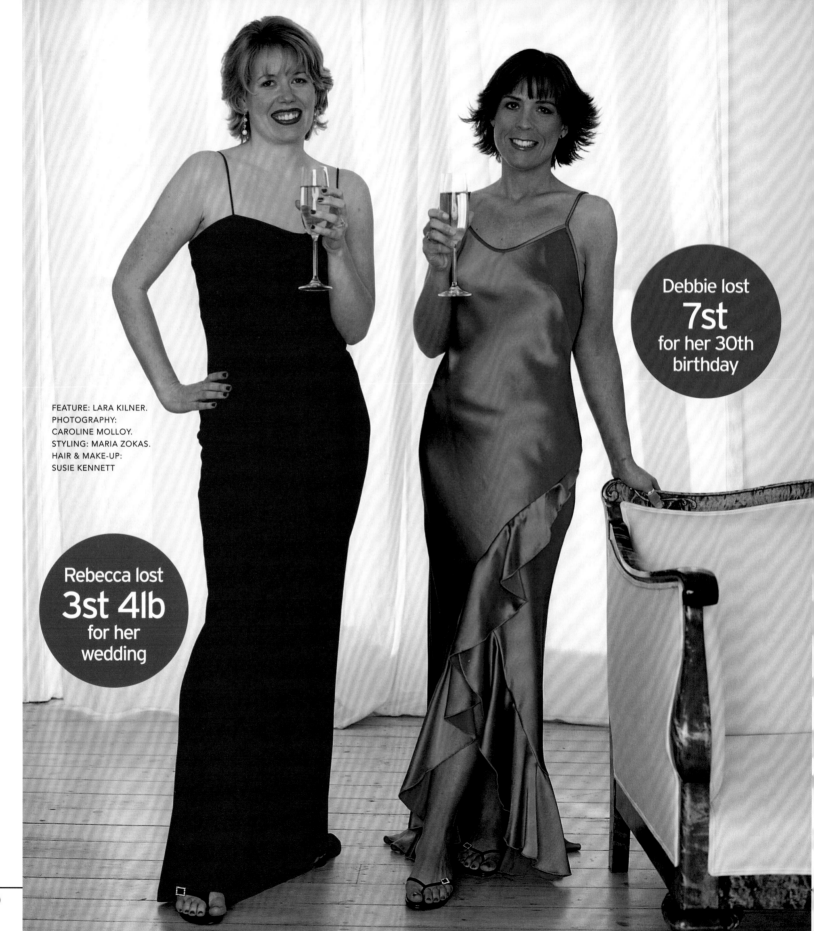

FEATURE: LARA KILNER.
PHOTOGRAPHY:
CAROLINE MOLLOY.
STYLING: MARIA ZOKAS.
HAIR & MAKE-UP:
SUSIE KENNETT

Debbie lost
7st
for her 30th
birthday

Rebecca lost
3st 4lb
for her
wedding

'We felt fantastic on the big day!'

One of the golden rules to slimming success is to set yourself a goal. And when you're on a weight-loss programme, a special occasion could be all it takes to get you thundering towards your target weight. Meet the readers who reached theirs – and changed their lives...

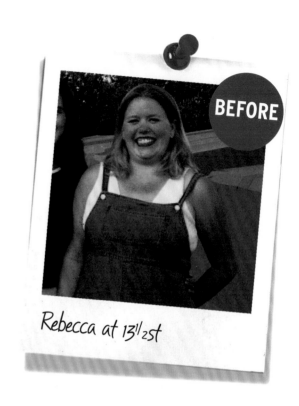

Rebecca at 13¹/₂st

Rebecca lost over 3st for her wedding to Matt

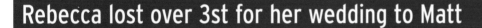

When did you start your weight loss plan?
'Matt proposed to me in a restaurant in Newquay on Millennium night and, once we started planning the wedding and looking at churches a year before the big day, I made a big promise to myself to lose my excess weight. Without the wedding as a focus, I don't think I would have lost as much as I did. I'm sure I would have got down to a size 14 and thought: 'I'm happy with this now', but having the wedding date to aim for gave me the drive to keep going with my diet and exercise plans.'

And did it make a difference to your big day...?
'It made a huge difference. I loved every minute of the day! I am quite shy but, because I had lost the weight, I wasn't that worried about being the centre of attention. I hated having my picture taken when I was bigger but, as it was, I didn't mind a bit – I even had a video camera filming me all day. And all my family and friends who hadn't seen me for a while couldn't believe how slim I was.'

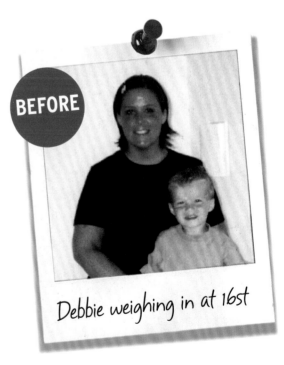

Debbie weighing in at 16st

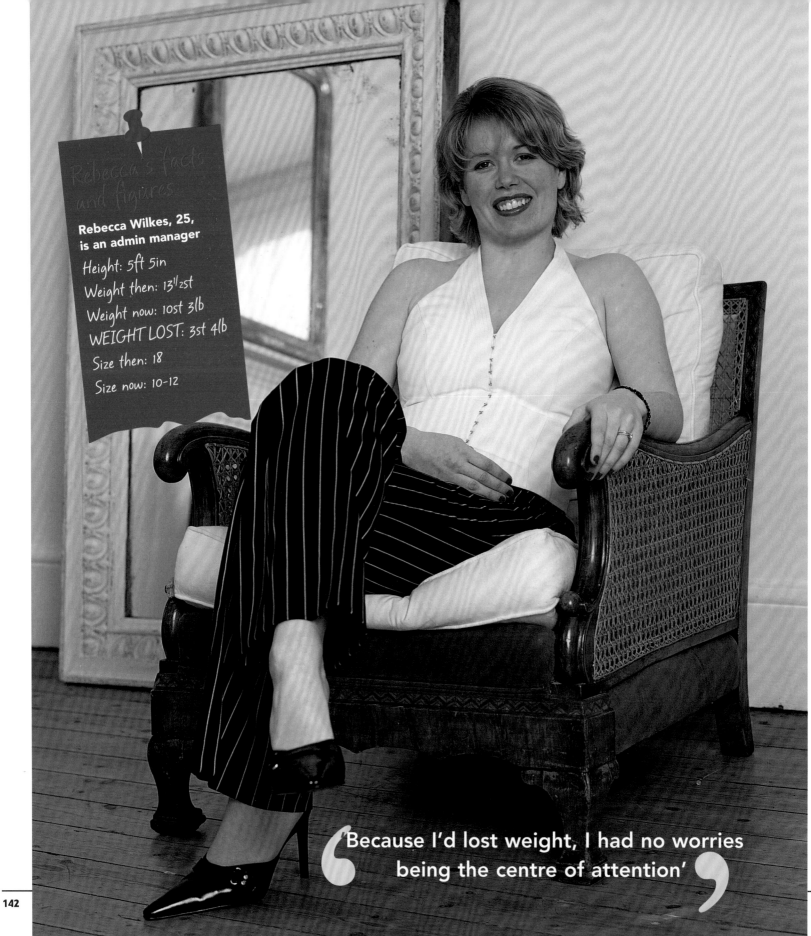

Rebecca's facts and figures

**Rebecca Wilkes, 25,
is an admin manager**

Height: 5ft 5in
Weight then: 13¹/₂st
Weight now: 10st 3lb
WEIGHT LOST: 3st 4lb
Size then: 18
Size now: 10-12

'Because I'd lost weight, I had no worries
being the centre of attention'

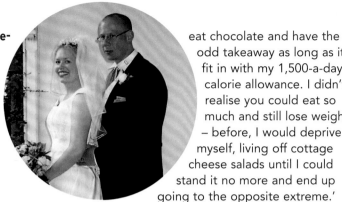

And then there's the slinky size-12 dress... 'The dress was a problem! I'd ordered it after I'd only lost a stone but, as I started to lose more weight, I had to have it taken in again every time I went for a fitting. I lost so much weight that eventually it had to be unpicked and remade.'

Your newly-slim figure must have made the honeymoon better, too...
'We went to the Bahamas and Florida and I wore a bikini for the first time in my life. I used to hate hot weather because of wearing less clothes, but now I can go on holiday without feeling self-conscious. I bought so many clothes for the honeymoon, I'd shoot myself if I put weight back on and couldn't wear them any more!'

The big question: how did you do it?
'I joined a slimming club, as I didn't think I could do it alone – I needed someone to keep an eye on me. I found counting calories easy because it was foods I'm used to. I could still

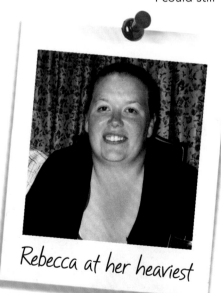

Rebecca at her heaviest

eat chocolate and have the odd takeaway as long as it fit in with my 1,500-a-day calorie allowance. I didn't realise you could eat so much and still lose weight – before, I would deprive myself, living off cottage cheese salads until I could stand it no more and end up going to the opposite extreme.'

So it's not the first time you've tried to lose weight, then?
'I'd tried half-heartedly before, but my weight didn't bother me enough then. I'd been chubby at school, and piled on more weight when I moved in with Matt, aged 19. We had bad habits – going to McDonald's for breakfast, and eating huge portions – whatever we cooked for dinner, I'd have half of it, however much there was. But my weight was never an issue for Matt or me then.

'I never thought I'd be this slim – six months on I'm still amazed! I got a new t-shirt last week just because the small size fit me – it wasn't even that nice!'

Did exercise play a big part in your impressive transformation?
'I've worked at a health club for two years and, when I first started, I didn't do any exercise. My colleagues are all fit and healthy and I'd feel self-conscious if I ate a lot. I'd just have a sandwich for lunch, but eat crisps and chocolate on the way home when no one could see.

'I'd never used the facilities at work, but it was easy for me to get fit when the wedding plans began. I used the gym once a week and did an aerobics class every Friday, which I still do. I also do body sculpting to tone up. My boss motivates me – she says she'll stop my wages if I back out of a class!'

What was the key to your success?
'Learning about food. I really educated myself – now I'm a pro at reading food labels. I have a cereal bar and a yoghurt for breakfast; a sandwich for lunch (without mayo or butter!); and fruit or yoghurt for an afternoon snack. Dinner will be something like chilli, with stacks of vegetables, followed by a snack-size chocolate bar.'

And I hear your new, healthy lifestyle rubbed off on a few other people...
'My mum came to the slimming club, which was a great support *and* she lost 10lb for her big day as mother of the bride! And as Matt was eating the healthy meals I was cooking, he lost 1½st! We were shadows of our former selves on the day!'

What did Matt make of his slim bride?
We were both really proud of me! It was the best day of my life. I can't imagine having photos of a day that I'd hated. I didn't realise how unhappy the excess weight made me until I got rid of it. Now I couldn't be happier.'

YOU CAN GET THE SHAPE YOU WANT FOR YOUR BIG DAY!

❑ **Visualise** the day, and how you will look and feel slimmed down
❑ **Plan** what you're going wear and the compliments you'll get!
❑ **Tell** close friends about your goal – but don't tell everyone. Enjoy the gasps, when people see how great you're looking.
❑ **Get support** from a slimming club to help reach your goal.
❑ **Keep it simple** – work out how many weeks until your big day. Aim to lose 2lb a week. If it's only two weeks, just think how fab you'll feel 4lb lighter!

Debbie, why did your looming 30th birthday spur you into action?

'I'd been overweight since childhood. Apart from having my son Bradley, now six, I felt hadn't achieved much.

'I didn't want to start a new decade as the same fat, miserable person. I felt a sense of urgency, like my life was being wasted. I realised there was no point being down about something I could change. Once I'd decided, I just did it.'

What made you stick to your goal?

'Anger to start with – I was furious I'd wasted so much of my life unhappy and overweight. So my 30th birthday drove me – and I never strayed from my diet.

'As the weight fell off I was driven by my happier outlook on life, and by my son. He's so proud of me, and really helped me, keeping me in check at the supermarket, and standing behind me when I was weighed at slimming club.

And what about the big day... how did you celebrate?

'When my birthday arrived I was 10st 2lb. I beamed all day! My sisters said we could do whatever I wanted so we went shopping and I tried on loads of size-12 clothes – just because I could! In the evening, we went for dinner. I was so high on my clothes shopping, I could hardly speak, let alone eat! I knew I could get much more happiness from my new outfits than from a dessert. Bradley celebrated too, lifting his apple juice to make a

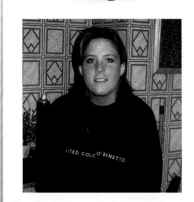

Debbie used to cover up

toast. Losing weight was my present to myself – that was all I needed. I felt complete. Now I'm looking forward to the rest of my life.'

Had you tried to lose weight before?

'I tried many diets, and took slimming tablets which made me feel peculiar and down. I yo-yo dieted, losing a couple of stone, then putting it back on, but I never got below 14st.

'Seven years ago, my mum died from lung cancer. For the six months she was ill, I barely ate. My marriage to Peter, Bradley's father, was breaking up and doctors thought I was having a breakdown. I lost over 6st, but knew this was an unhealthy way to lose it. But not long after mum died I turned to food again. I put the weight back on quickly, plus even more!

How did you turn things around and make this diet a success?

'Simple – I joined a slimming club and followed a 1,500-calorie-a-day diet.

'I was amazed at how much I could eat. Eating four Weetabix for breakfast stopped me snacking until lunch when I'd have a huge tuna salad. Dinner was chicken with loads of veggies. Now I cook lots of types of veg each day and Bradley and I love cabbage!

'I marked my birthday in big red letters on the calender and thought every day about how I'd feel if I was still overweight on the big day – that kept me going. I weighed food, and wrote down everything I'd eaten – that stopped me binge-ing.'

Were you as virtuous with exercise?

'No, I can't exercise. I was diag-

nosed at age 16 with the rare medical condition myasthenia gravis, which means I have very weak muscles. My medication stops me collapsing in a heap after any slight exertion, and stops it getting worse, but it's tough. It feels like I'm trying to run through a swimming pool, working against resistance. I'd love to go to the gym, but I can't even walk for too long.'

Having that obstacle makes losing weight an even bigger achievement. Do you blame the condition for making you overweight?

'Not being active can't have helped, but I don't blame it. I was big because I ate too much. My life revolved around food – I'd plan what I could eat next.

'I was at least 2st heavier than my schoolmates. It made me miserable, but I didn't try to change it. I'd feel depressed, but then my mum would dish up a shepherd's pie and I'd think: 'Lovely!' and tuck in. Long after leaving school, things didn't change. In a typical day I'd eat buttered toast for breakfast, peanut butter and banana sandwiches with crisps and chocolate at lunch, and an unhealthy dinner – everything with chips or big piles of mash, or takeaways. I'd snack on cakes and family-size bags of crisps – there were times when I'd eat two or three family bags of Doritos, and two or three Twix bars – never just one. I'd get up in the night and have Coco Pops – sometimes three times in a night. And I'd even put sugar on veg!

What's different now?

'I feel healthy. When I look at fatty foods I think about what they could do to me. You only get one body and it has to last a lifetime – finally I'm treating mine well.

'I've broken my comfort-eating cycle. I was overeating because I was fat, and I was fat because I was overeating. But now I know I'm never going back.'

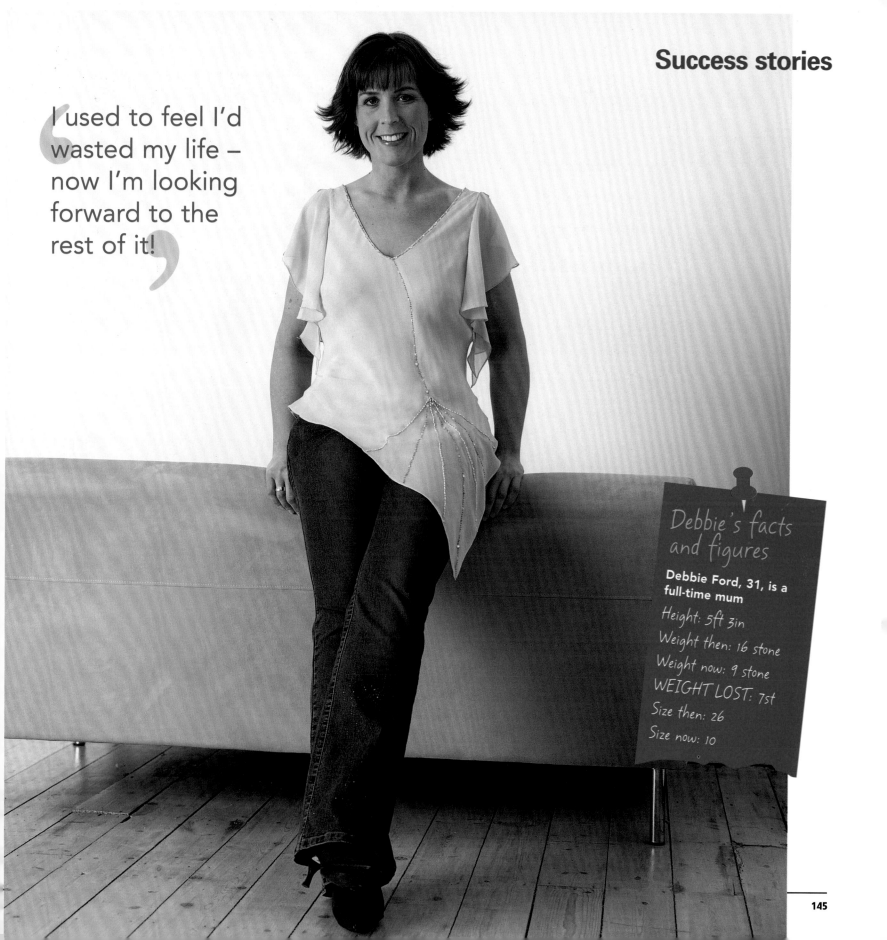

"I used to feel I'd wasted my life – now I'm looking forward to the rest of it!"

Debbie's facts and figures

Debbie Ford, 31, is a full-time mum

Height: 5ft 3in

Weight then: 16 stone

Weight now: 9 stone

WEIGHT LOST: 7st

Size then: 26

Size now: 10

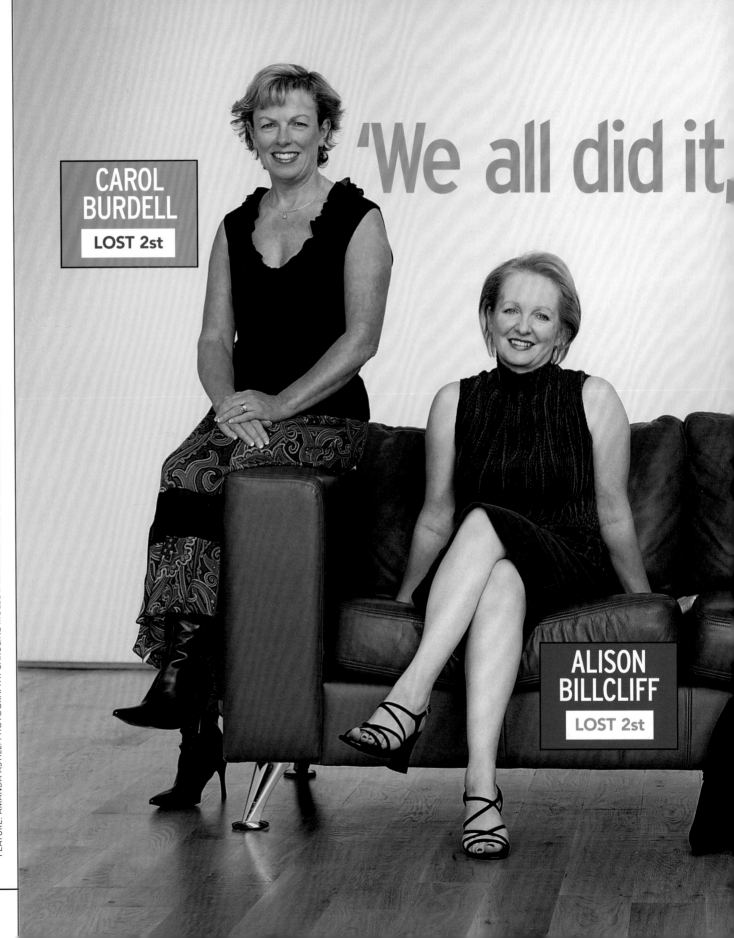

CAROL BURDELL

LOST 2st

'We all did it,

ALISON BILLCLIFF

LOST 2st

so can you'

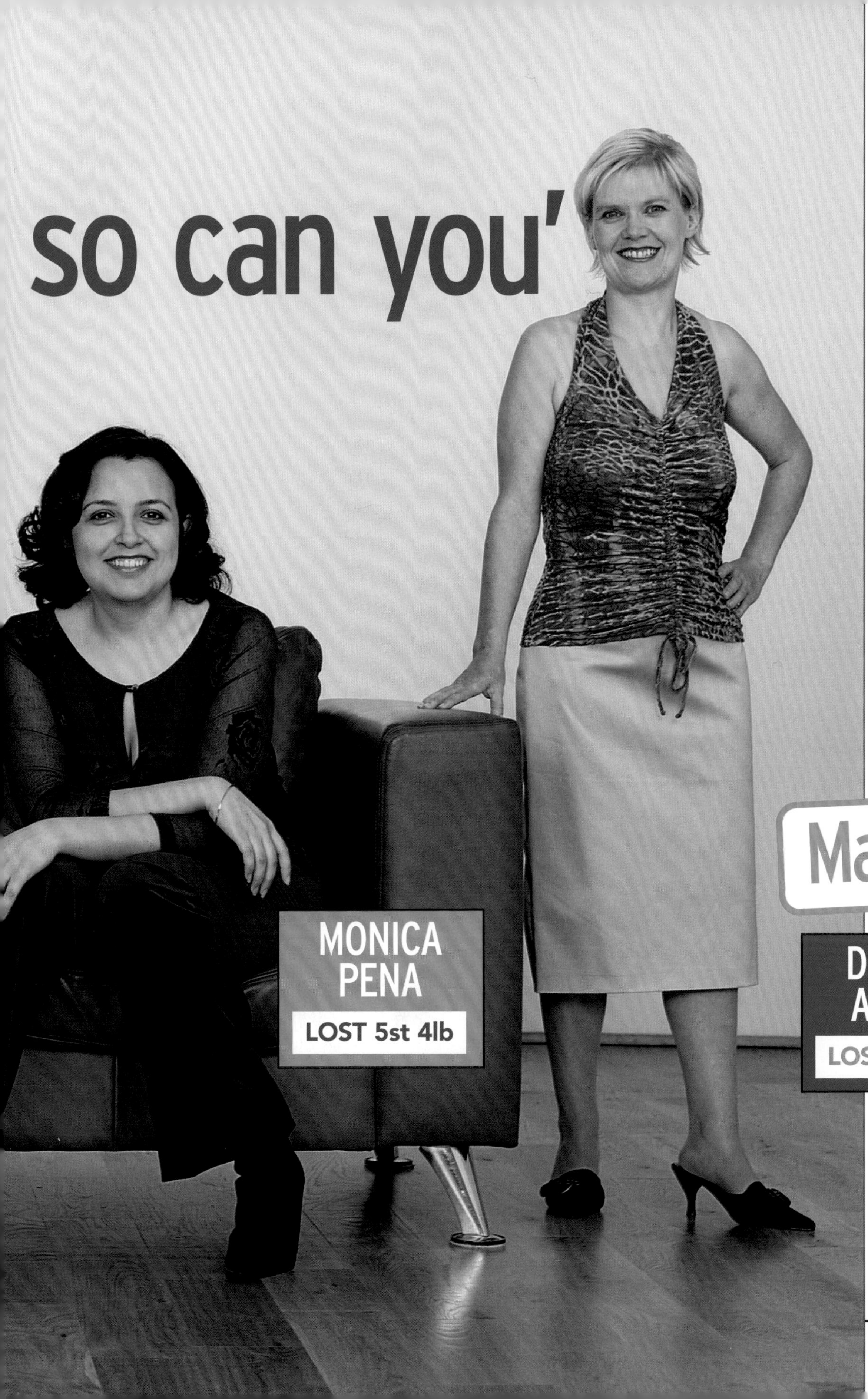

On New Year's Eve, these four women each vowed to lose weight – between them they're now 13st lighter

Make it happen!

MONICA PENA

LOST 5st 4lb

DEBBIE ABBOT

LOST 3st 9lb

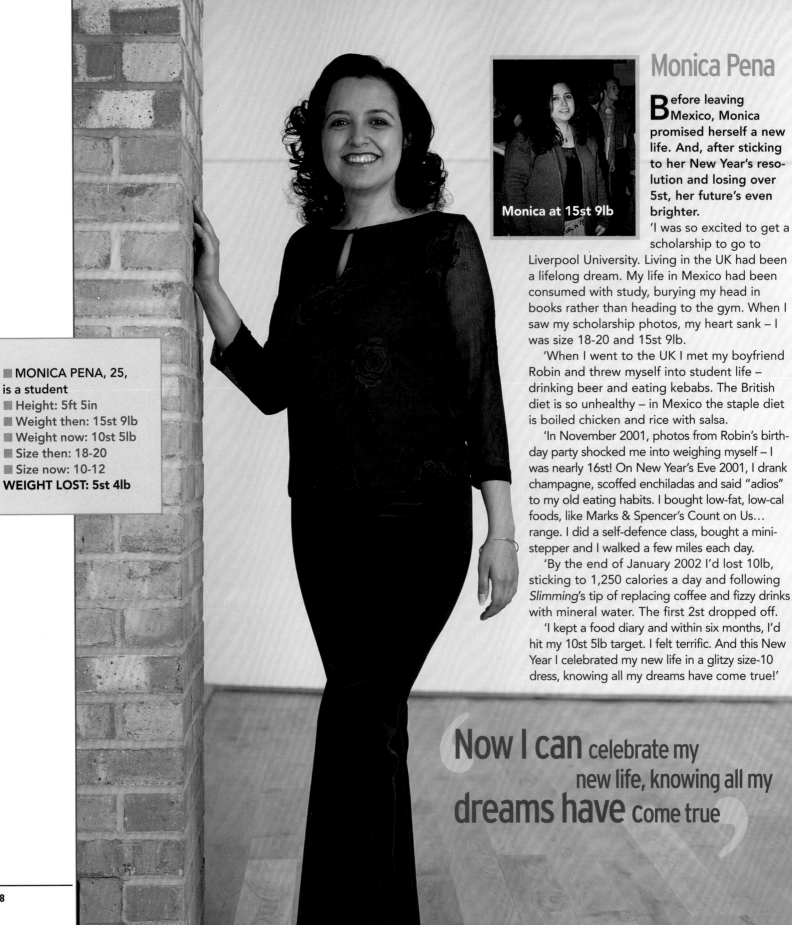

Monica Pena

Before leaving Mexico, Monica promised herself a new life. And, after sticking to her New Year's resolution and losing over 5st, her future's even brighter.

Monica at 15st 9lb

'I was so excited to get a scholarship to go to Liverpool University. Living in the UK had been a lifelong dream. My life in Mexico had been consumed with study, burying my head in books rather than heading to the gym. When I saw my scholarship photos, my heart sank – I was size 18-20 and 15st 9lb.

'When I went to the UK I met my boyfriend Robin and threw myself into student life – drinking beer and eating kebabs. The British diet is so unhealthy – in Mexico the staple diet is boiled chicken and rice with salsa.

'In November 2001, photos from Robin's birthday party shocked me into weighing myself – I was nearly 16st! On New Year's Eve 2001, I drank champagne, scoffed enchiladas and said "adios" to my old eating habits. I bought low-fat, low-cal foods, like Marks & Spencer's Count on Us… range. I did a self-defence class, bought a mini-stepper and I walked a few miles each day.

'By the end of January 2002 I'd lost 10lb, sticking to 1,250 calories a day and following *Slimming*'s tip of replacing coffee and fizzy drinks with mineral water. The first 2st dropped off.

'I kept a food diary and within six months, I'd hit my 10st 5lb target. I felt terrific. And this New Year I celebrated my new life in a glitzy size-10 dress, knowing all my dreams have come true!'

■ **MONICA PENA, 25, is a student**
■ Height: 5ft 5in
■ Weight then: 15st 9lb
■ Weight now: 10st 5lb
■ Size then: 18-20
■ Size now: 10-12
WEIGHT LOST: 5st 4lb

'Now I can celebrate my new life, knowing all my dreams have come true'

'I'm lighter now than I was when I got pregnant, something I never thought possible'

Alison Billcliff

Depressed at celebrating the Millennium in a dress she'd worn during pregnancy, Alison resolved to get in shape by joining a slimming club, and lost 2st.

'I raised a toast to the New Year at my mother-in-law's champagne supper, but my heart wasn't in it – I couldn't ignore my size.

'When I became a mother again at 41, I didn't worry about my weight. The pounds had dropped off after my first two, but this time it was a different story. I'd hoped to wear a figure-hugging dress for the Millennium, but instead saw in the New Year overweight, despondent and dressed in a frumpy outfit. Making the resolution to lose weight was actually a big relief. "This is my year to be slim," I told myself. A neighbour had lost a lot of weight at a slimming club, so I decided to go along with her. Joining the club made my resolution seem real.

'I was convinced I ate healthily but my size-16 clothes said otherwise. Salads were doused in full-fat mayo, served with chunks of bread and washed down with wine. My husband and I liked going out for meals, relaxing on holiday with a glass of beer and cuddling up at home with a stash of chocolate.

'The club was a revelation – I was amazed at how easy the diet was. I stuck to chicken salads, minus the mayo and bread, and didn't have to change my lifestyle at all – just cut out the little extras. Nothing was forbidden and I ate and drank everything in moderation, sticking to my 1,500 calorie quota.

'January can be depressing for some people, but my New Year's resolution made me positive about the future. By the end of the month I'd lost a stone. That gave me the incentive to lose another. In fact, I'm lighter now than I was when I got pregnant, something I never thought possible!'

ALISON BILLCLIFF, 44, is a medical secretary
- Height: 5ft 2in
- Weight then: 10½st
- Weight now: 8½st
- Size then: 16
- Size now: 10
WEIGHT LOST: 2st

Alison at 10½st

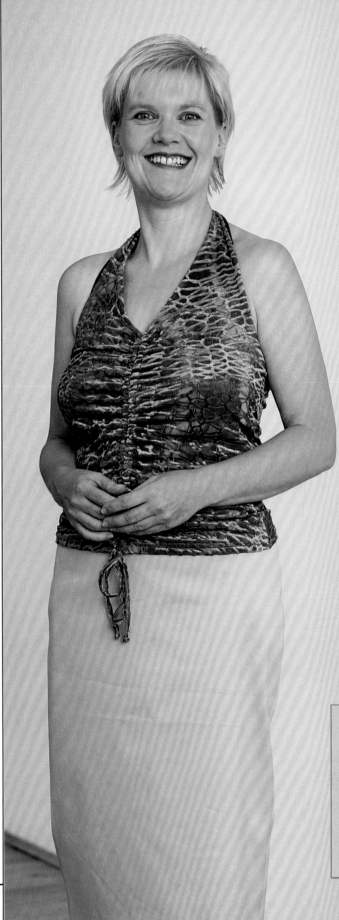

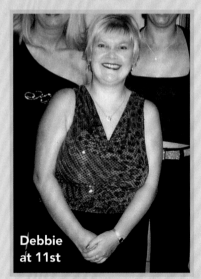

Debbie
at 11st

Debbie Abbot

When Debbie spent New Year's Eve 2001 stuck on the sofa scoffing chocolate, she vowed next year would be different. After losing 3½st, she spent last New Year partying in a glamorous size-8 outfit.

'Shopping for something to wear to my office party, I'd reduced my criteria to a simple: "Does it fit?" And I was happy with the black velvet skirt and red sequin top I'd bought – until I saw the photos. Red sequins and that chest – hello?

'Six years ago, my husband died in a motorbike accident. I spent most nights watching TV with my son, Daniel, bingeing on crisps. I couldn't be bothered to cook and often had takeaways. I piled on 3st – at 11st, I was far too heavy. I'd say: "Tomorrow I'll go on a diet," but I never did.

'On New Year's Eve 2001, Daniel and I watched TV. I flopped into bed just after midnight – depressed. As a mum in my 30s, I felt my life was ticking away. I had to lose weight to get back my self-respect.

'I resolved to join a slimming club and start living. I threw out junk snacks and filled the fridge with healthy foods – grilled chicken breasts were my saviour. Sticking to 1,200 calories a day, I lost 12lb by the end of January 2002. In six months I hit my target 7st 5lb. The other day our window cleaner yelled out: "It's the incredible shrinking woman!"

'I've now joined a gym and take Tai Kwondo classes. I'm also doing an accounting course. Losing weight has given me the inspiration to change my life. This New Year I partied and wore a sexy outfit. This is the new me!'

Losing the weight has given me the inspiration to change my life

- ■ **DEBBIE ABBOT, 35, is a civil service finance officer**
- ■ Height: 4ft 10½in
- ■ Weight then: 11st
- ■ Weight now: 7st 5lb
- ■ Size then: 18
- ■ Size now: 8
- **TOTAL WEIGHT LOST: 3st 9lb**

'My resolution was a major turning point – I may be 50 but I'm not frumpy'

Carol Burdell

Feeling fat, frumpy and fed up with festive cheer, Carol gave up booze for New Year. Now 2st lighter, she feels years younger.

'"Don't worry, love, we all put on a bit at 50," my husband, Len, assured me. It was New Year's Eve 2001 and we were at the golf club party, enjoying the buffet.

'After going on HRT at 48, the pounds piled on. I was sick of hearing: "It's fine at your age." It wasn't fine, because I wasn't fine – I was miserable. Sick of festive booze and buffet binges, I made a New Year's resolution: I couldn't go on getting bigger – I didn't want to be fat, frumpy and 50.

'My main downfall was drinking – I enjoy a glass of wine and the nibble factor that goes with it. So I went teetotal for January. I joined a slimming club and cut my calories to 1,250 a day. It was easier than I expected – no faddy dieting. I was so focused, even giving up alcohol was no problem – seeing the pounds drop off increased my resolve. By the end of January 2002 I'd lost ½st. After losing another 1½st, I'd hit my target.

'Now I love shopping with Hannah, my 19-year-old, knowing I can fit into trendy clothes too. I'm 50 but I'm not frumpy. My resolution was a major turning point. And this New Year I wasn't glued to the buffet!'

- ■ **CAROL BURDELL, 50, is a medical secretary**
- ■ Height: 5ft
- ■ Weight before: 10½st
- ■ Weight now: 8½st
- ■ Size before: 14
- ■ Size now: 10
- **WEIGHT LOST: 2st**

Carol at 10½st

I shed 5st
against the odds!

Her health was against her, but Linda Thomas still managed to lose 5st in time to celebrate her silver wedding anniversary

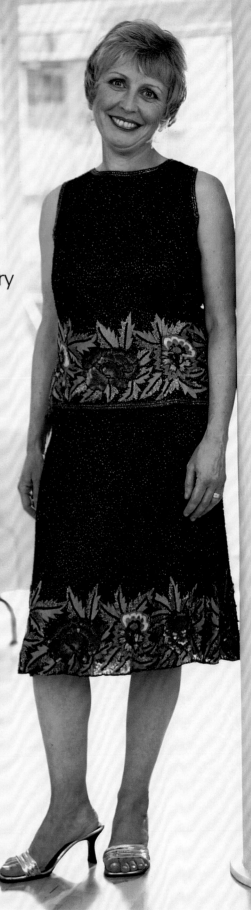

FEATURE: CATHERINE FRANCIS. PHOTOGRAPHY: DAVE ANTHONY. HAIR & MAKE-UP: SUSIE KENNETT. STYLING: MARIA ZOKAS

Tipping the scales at more than 13st and with her silver wedding anniversary on the horizon, Linda Thomas decided it was time to take action. And she wasn't about to let the fact that she had an underactive thyroid hold her back. 'I recently read a magazine article that said it's almost impossible to lose weight if you have an underactive thyroid,' says Linda. 'I felt like writing in to say that it was rubbish! It might be harder, but it can be done. I'm proof of that.'

Linda's facts & figures

LINDA THOMAS, 48, IS A LAB ASSISTANT

Height:	**5ft 1in**
Weight then:	**13st 1lb**
Weight now:	**8½st**
WEIGHT LOST:	**4st 8lb**
Size then:	**20**
Size now:	**10-12**

When did you first start to have a problem with your weight?
I've been overweight most of my life. As a child, I wasn't slim. We ate healthily – just too much. Mum always kept the cupboards full, and I ate because it was there. My sister and one of my brothers are heavy, though my parents weren't, and my other brother is like a piece of string!

In my teens, I weighed about 10st, but I wasn't concerned. I was a bit self-conscious – I never wore sleeveless clothes – but no one treated me badly. I was no shrinking violet and I had an active social life.

At 21, I married Dave, an HGV driver. I weighed about 10st 3lb, and looking at photos of myself in my big soppy wedding dress, I think: 'My goodness, I looked like a big fat fairy!' But I didn't think so at the time and I loved every minute of my big day. Four years later, along came our daughter, Rebecca, who's now 23.

Did you put on weight during your pregnancy with Rebecca?
Not particularly. But I gave up work to look after her and often sat with other mums, chatting and eating biscuits. By the time Rebecca was six, I weighed 11st. One day, I looked in the mirror and thought, 'Goodness!'. I decided to do something about it, but I must have taken leave of my senses because I almost stopped eating altogether. My weight plummeted to 8st, but I looked – and felt – tired and unhealthy.

The weight soon piled back on – and more. Two years later, I weighed 12st, and I stayed at that weight for a few years until I stopped smoking. My mum said: 'It's better to be overweight than a smoker', so I chose biscuits and chocolate over cigarettes and my clothes soon got even tighter.

BEFORE: *'I couldn't face the thought of wearing a swimsuit in public'*

AFTER: *'I bought two bikinis for our holiday in Cyprus this year'*

When did you find out that you had a thyroid problem?

Five years ago I visited my GP because I was tired and having difficulty concentrating. A blood test showed I had an underactive thyroid. My doctor explained that it makes you put on weight – although I knew I also ate too much. I was prescribed thyroxine and within days I felt 100% better. In just weeks, I lost ½st without even trying. At that point I was content, and my weight didn't bother me too much.

What changed that?

Pure vanity! It was October 1999, and the following year would be Rebecca's 21st birthday, our silver wedding anniversary, and the Millennium celebrations. I just thought: 'I don't want to be fat anymore.'

A colleague and I joined a slimming club. But I have to admit that I checked it out first to make sure we wouldn't be the biggest people there!

At my first weigh-in, the group leader told me I weighed 13st 1lb. 'I think your scales are wrong, dear,' I said. I tried three sets of scales before I accepted the horrible truth.

What changes did you make to the way you ate?

I stopped snacking and made sure I always ate a good breakfast of cereal or toast and some fruit. Throughout the day I ate lots of fruit and vegetables, and when I was grocery shopping I made sure I read the fat and calorie contents of the foods I bought. But I didn't deprive myself and enjoyed treats, like a glass of wine. And it paid off – I managed to lose a steady 2lb a week. My colleague lost heart and stopped going, but I never fell off the wagon or gave into temptation.

After a few months, my weight loss slowed to 1lb a week. I started to feel a little despondent. It's at times like that you really need the encouragement of a club. The ritual humiliation – sorry, weekly weigh-in! – kept me on the straight and narrow.

When I lost 3½st, the club leader put me on a podium and asked me to pick up an old metal sewing machine – I could barely lift it. She then announced that the machine weighed 50lb – the same amount as I'd lost!

Were your family and friends encouraging?

My husband Dave always told me not to worry about my weight – which is kind, but not very inspirational. I told everybody at work that I was slimming and I was always jumping on our big industrial scales, so I knew they'd guess something was going on! Everyone was really encouraging and expected weekly updates on my progress.

Did you do any exercise?

I'm not a natural exerciser, and don't really like classes. But I walk to work and am always on the go – according to my pedometer, I manage to clock up 3½ miles a day! Dave and I now go swimming once a week, too.

How long did it take you to reach target?

When the club leader suggested 9½st as my goal, I thought, 'In your dreams'. But within six months, I'd hit my target! I continued losing weight until I got down to 8½st, less than two months later.

I'm still mentally counting calories – my brain's like a little calculator. It's a good habit to get into, though.

How was your silver wedding anniversary?

Lovely – we invited friends for dinner and I felt fabulous in a size-12 dress. People who hadn't seen me for a while were amazed.

Dave maintains that my weight makes no difference to him. He's known me fat, he's known me slim and he's always loved me whatever my shape. I think he's secretly chuffed I'm not big anymore, but he'd never admit it because I'd be mortified.

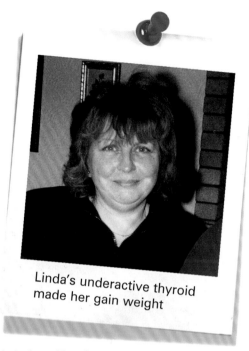

Linda's underactive thyroid made her gain weight

What's the best thing about being slim?

I feel so much healthier and I'm much more confident. I'd never have considered swimming before – I couldn't face the thought of wearing a swimsuit in public. And I've always loved clothes, but there's more for me to choose from now. I bought two bikinis for our holiday in Cyprus this year. I'd never worn a bikini in my life, but I didn't think twice about it. It was great!

THE THYROID LOWDOWN

Slimming's **resident GP Dr Roger Henderson says**: 'The thyroid gland, situated in the neck, produces hormones that regulate metabolism. Insufficient hormone production leads to a lower metabolism, a symptom of which is weight gain.

'The main cause is an auto-immune inflammation of the thyroid, where the body's immune system attacks its own tissues. It can also be caused by certain medicines, or excessive amounts of kelp supplements. Other symptoms include constipation, lethargy and dry skin and hair, so if you suspect you may have an underactive thyroid, visit your GP.

'If you have an underactive thyroid, you'll be treated with the replacement hormone thyroxine, which will normalise your metabolism and make it easier for you to lose weight.'

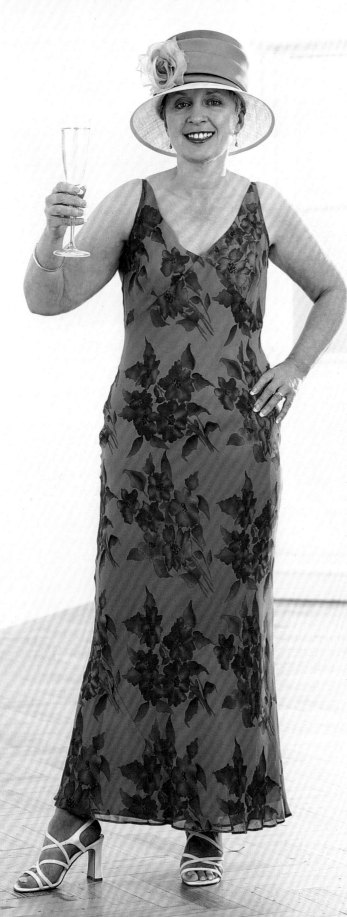

I dropped 5 for a family

Desperate to be slim for her stepdaughter's big day, Helen Walters tackled her bad eating habits and lost nearly 6st…

It should have been a joyful moment for the whole family. But when her stepdaughter Sarah announced that she was getting married, all Helen Walters felt was panic. 'For years, I'd avoided going out because I felt too ashamed of my appearance,' says Helen. 'But I just couldn't miss Sarah's wedding day. I felt miserable, desperate – and guilty for not being happier about her big day. But I had to be honest with myself – I was dreading going to her wedding because of how I looked.'

Hiding away because of her weight was something Helen had done for most of her life. 'I was always the chubby one of the family,' she recalls. 'I had a very sweet tooth. My mum couldn't understand why I was overweight, because I didn't appear to eat that much. But I was secretly spending my pocket money on sweets, cakes and chocolates. I'd even spend my bus fare on sweets and walk to school.'

Throughout her teenage years, Helen's weight gradually increased until, at 17, she weighed in at 13st 3lb. 'My weight affected everything,' she remembers. 'People weren't unkind to me, but I felt really awful about myself. I tried to keep up with fashion, but I thought I looked ridiculous in trendy clothes. All my friends had boyfriends,

but I never did. And PE lessons were sheer hell – I'd do anything I could to get out of them.'

Desperate to lose weight, at 17 Helen embarked on a crash diet. But her desire to be slim spiralled dangerously out of control. 'I starved myself,' admits Helen. 'I lived on black coffee plus one yoghurt and one lemon a day – which I'd just peel and eat. I was so paranoid about gaining any weight, I wouldn't even take an aspirin. My mother was so worried that, in desperation, she crushed vitamin tablets and put them in my coffee. My weight plummeted to under 6st and I was diagnosed with anorexia. I was in and out of hospital for about a year, and I didn't have a period for a couple of years.'

Things improved when, at 19, Helen found herself a boyfriend, Tony, and they got married a year later. Feeling more content with life, she managed to beat her anorexia and put on an impressive 6st. But her unhealthy relationship with food wasn't over. 'When it came to food, it was all or nothing,' recalls Helen. 'I was either pigging out, or starving myself. I couldn't steer a middle course. Throughout my 20s, I swung between 13st and 8st. Each time, I'd starve myself and feel elated at my success. But once I hit target, I'd start bingeing and the

dress sizes
wedding

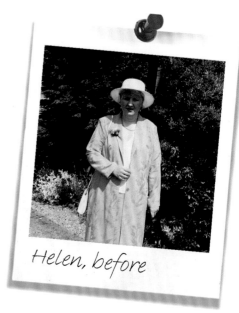

Helen, before

weight would pile back on.

'My weight wasn't an issue at all for Tony but, again, I kept my bingeing secret. I had a stash of sweets and cakes, and I'd regularly eat four or five chocolate bars in one sitting. It never even occurred to me that exercising would help stabilise my weight.'

Although Helen never slipped back into anorexia, the illness came back to haunt her when she and Tony started trying for a baby. She managed to conceive twice, but both were ectopic pregnancies, where the foetus develops in the

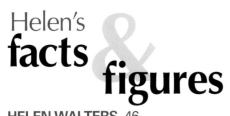

Helen's facts & figures

HELEN WALTERS, 46, IS AN ADMIN MANAGER

Height:	5ft 3in
Weight then:	15st 10lb
Weight now:	9st 12lb
WEIGHT LOST:	5st 12lb
Size then:	22
Size now:	12

fallopian tube. The foetus, and usually the tube, have to be removed to save the mother's life.

'I was devastated, as doctors believed my anorexia may have robbed me of the chance to have children, although we can't be sure that was actually the cause,' Helen recalls. 'I felt guilty and wondered what I had to live for – and I comforted myself with food.'

They never did get to have any children and, when she was 30, Helen and Tony split up. Feeling emotional and lacking self-confidence, Helen then embarked on another crash diet, getting down to 9½st – but once again, her weight soon started increasing.

'At 33, I met my second husband, Robert, through work,' says Helen. 'I weighed about 11½st, but Robert made me feel attractive and we soon moved in together. He never commented on my weight, but my increasing size meant I could never face going out, or on holiday. If Robert was invited to dinner with his boss, I'd make some excuse not to go. I felt ugly and frumpy, and could never seem to find anything nice to wear. Robert said he didn't want to go out without me, so he was stuck in all the time as well. He was frustrated, and I felt really awful for spoiling his fun.'

At 35, Helen decided to quit smoking. But she found it tough giving up her 30-a-day habit, and snacked on sweets and biscuits instead. Her weight soon reached 13st.

'Then, at 38, I started an early menopause, which may have happened due to my previous

gynaecological problems,' says Helen. 'After I started taking hormone replacement therapy (HRT), my weight seemed to increase even faster. In less than a year, I weighed over 14st. My doctor didn't show me much sympathy, though, and told me I should just eat less and exercise. I was tempted to stop taking the HRT altogether, but my GP warned me about the risk of osteoporosis if I did, so I just learned to live with it.'

After living together for seven years, Helen and Robert decided to tie the knot in 1997. Keen to lose weight for her big day, Helen once again slipped back into bad eating habits. Existing on just a yoghurt or piece of fruit for lunch, and meat and two veg for dinner, she lost 3st, taking her down to 11st. 'But I felt constantly weak and cold,' she admits, 'and I picked up every virus going around.' Once married, Helen was straight back to the biscuit tin, and in three years, her weight soared to over 15st.

It was in May 2001, when Helen was at her heaviest weight of 15st 10lb, that Robert's daughter Sarah announced she was getting married the following year. 'Desperate not to feel fat at her wedding, I once again started dieting like mad,' says Helen. 'But this time, I couldn't shift the weight. In two months, I lost just a couple of pounds and I finally came to my senses about the way that I was trying to lose weight. I realised yo-yo dieting had messed up my metabolism. And, of course, you

Does HRT make you gain weight?

GP DR ROGER HENDERSON SAYS:
'Many women are concerned about gaining weight on HRT (hormone replacement therapy). But research shows that HRT itself doesn't cause an increase in weight. However, it might increase your appetite, particularly if you feel better in yourself because of the treatment, so pay extra attention to what you're eating and be sure to take regular exercise, as Helen was advised to. Interestingly, though, HRT has been shown to alter the distribution of weight on the body, to the hips and thighs rather than the abdomen. It's also worth noting, of course, that 45 per cent of women put on weight during their 50s and 60s – whether they're taking HRT or not.

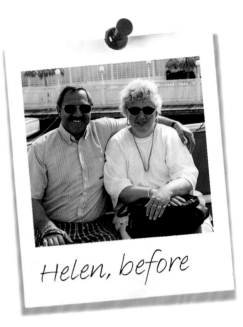

Helen, before

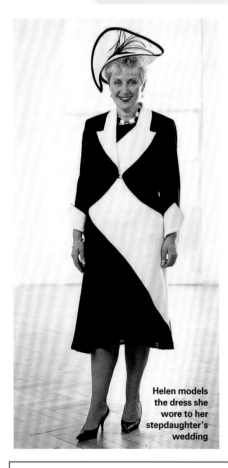

Helen models the dress she wore to her stepdaughter's wedding

don't lose weight as easily when you're older. I didn't know what to do next. Robert came to the rescue, though. 'He knew he'd have trouble getting me to the wedding if I didn't lose weight,' Helen says, 'so he convinced me that exercise and a healthy diet was the only way to slim.'

Despite a lifetime of avoiding exercise at all costs, Helen was so desperate she decided to finally give it a go. But she just couldn't face the gym. 'Robert saw a treadmill in a catalogue,' recalls Helen. 'At £350, it certainly wasn't cheap. But he offered to pay half, and we agreed to pay it off over six months.

'We set the treadmill up in the garage and I starting walking on it for just 10 minutes a day, at 5km an hour. It was hard work at first but I stuck to it. Each week, I increased my time by 10%. A few months later, I was walking for 30 minutes a day. Then I gradually increased the speed, and set the treadmill on a slight incline to make it harder.'

Helen began to shed a steady 1lb-2lb a week. After two months, her clothes started to feel a bit looser, which really encouraged her to keep going. 'And knowing the treadmill was costing us £35 each month made me think I'd better make good use of it!' she laughs. Helen's new exercise regime also helped her

stick to a healthy diet for the first time in her life. A typical daily menu was now two slices of wholemeal toast with Marmite for breakfast; fruit for a mid-morning snack; a lunch of soup and a roll; meat and vegetables or spaghetti bolognese for dinner; and a low-calorie chocolate drink before bed.

'Exercising made me more relaxed about my eating habits,' Helen says. 'If I had a few treats, I knew I'd still lose weight. Even Christmas and holidays were fine – if I put on a few pounds, I'd just get back on the treadmill, and the weight would come off.'

When Helen got bored with working out on her own, Robert set up a TV in the garage so she could stride along while watching her favourite soap operas. And he encouraged her to keep going even when she didn't feel like it.

'Robert also spent £70 on some really accurate weighing scales for me,' says Helen. 'Some scales can be changeable, and you can become discouraged because of this. But these displayed my weight to the nearest ¼lb, so I could see when I'd lost even a small amount.

'I recorded my weight loss on a progress chart, which kept me motivated, and I was also encouraged by the real life success stories I read in *Slimming* every month. The magazine was also great for keeping me informed of new diet foods on the market, which stopped me getting bored with what I was eating.'

BEFORE: *'It never even occurred to me that exercising would help me lose weight'*   **AFTER:** *'I'm glad I started working out because now I really love it and actually look forward to it'*

Success stories

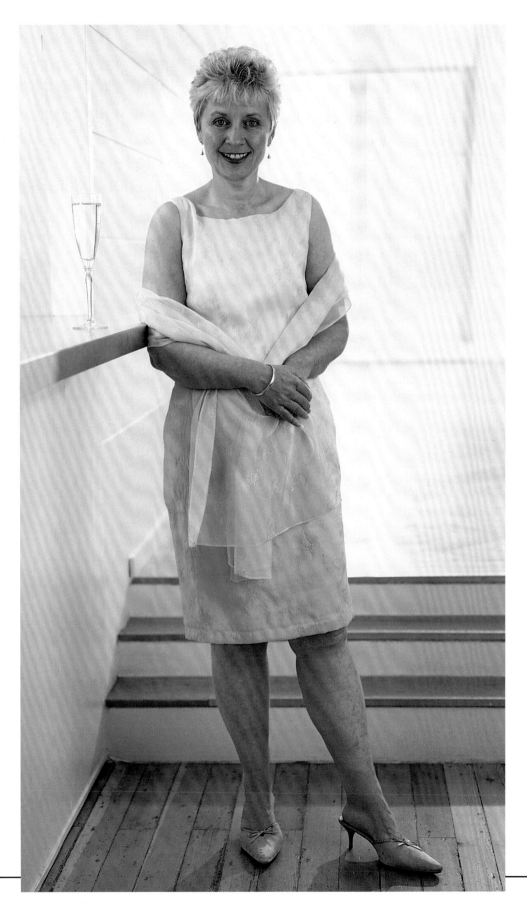

Helen reached her target weight of 9st 12lb in May – the very week of Sarah's wedding. 'I was thrilled,' she says. 'I bought a size-12 black and white dress, with a bolero jacket, which I felt – and looked – great in. And instead of dreading the big day, I really looked forward to it. The wedding was lovely and, rather than trying to blend into the background like I always had in the past, I had the confidence to talk to everyone – lots of people commented on how nice I looked. I really enjoyed myself and I'd love to do it all again! Robert had a wonderful day too, and I know he felt very proud of what I'd achieved.'

'I never believed exercise could speed up my metabolism and make such a difference to losing weight – but it really does,' enthuses Helen. 'Plus, I'm glad I started working out because now I really love it. Being slim has given me the confidence to meet new people. And I feel healthier than ever – I even sleep far better now that I'm fit and I don't have night sweats any more. Robert's much happier too. He always loved me, but he admits he finds me more attractive now, and he enjoys the busy new social life we've built up together.

'I can't believe I abused my body for so long. Now I've found out how to be fit and healthy, I'll keep exercising and eating sensibly – and I'm determined to keep the weight off for life.'

Helen's exercise tips

- If you don't like going to a gym, invest in an exercise bike, treadmill or rowing machine to use in the privacy of your own home. Shelling out good money for it will make you more likely to use it.
- Choose a convenient time to exercise that you find easy to stick to. I do half an hour as soon as I get home from work, and it's become an easy routine – in fact, I even look forward to getting home in the evening because of it!
- If you get bored, watch TV or listen to music while you exercise. That way, you'll hardly notice you're working out.
- Promise yourself a treat for all your hard work – a low-calorie chocolate drink is just the job for me.

Now I feel great in a bikini

Annamarie Teague used to dread wearing summer clothes. But now after losing nearly 4st, she can't wait to put on her bikini…

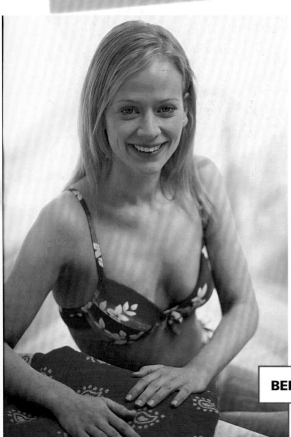

Annamarie, before

Coming from a large family, mealtimes at Annamarie Teague's house were a time for the whole family to come together and enjoy themselves – and that meant munching their way through huge portions and enormous stodgy puddings. No surprise, then, that Annamarie developed a sweet tooth.

'Being the youngest of seven kids, I got spoilt,' remembers Annamarie. 'Mum always fussed over me, saying, "You need to eat up if you want to grow into a big, strong girl." And my three brothers and three sisters always scraped their leftovers onto my plate.'

Although the rest of the family remained slim, at only 5ft tall Annamarie couldn't get away with carrying any extra weight. And after falling pregnant at 17, her size spiralled out of control.

It was only the thought of having to wear a bikini on a glamorous holiday in Ibiza in 2000 that pulled her back from the edge…

Did your weight problems make your teenage years tough?
Being a chubby teenager was no fun, and I experienced first-hand how cruel children can be. I tried to shrug off taunts of 'Miss Piggy' and 'fat cow', but inside I felt hurt and would cry myself to sleep at night. I dreaded the summer months – the thought of peeling off those big winter clothes and showing some flesh brought me out in a cold sweat. And having to run around in a little A-line skirt and T-shirt for outdoor PE lessons was a nightmare, so I'd forge sick notes to get out of it. These days, I really enjoy sport, and regret missing out on all those summer activities as a teenager, such as rounders, rowing and canoeing.

What about boyfriends?
At the age of 15, when I weighed about 10st, I met my current boyfriend, Amar – although to start with, we were just good friends. I didn't like eating in front of him – or in front of anyone else with whom I wasn't completely comfortable – so I saved my binges for when I was alone at home. If we were out somewhere and Amar wanted to have something to eat, I wouldn't have anything, even if I was starving – I didn't want people staring at me and thinking that I was too big to be eating a burger. Then, one day, I was visiting Amar's family and his mum ordered a pizza. I knew that if I didn't have some, I'd look silly – not to mention a bit neurotic – so I just tucked in. Grabbing that slice of pizza became a turning point in our relationship – I realised how comfortable I felt with Amar. I knew we'd make a great couple, and we soon stopped being just good friends…

So when did your weight start to become a real problem?
When I left school at the age of 16, a size 14 and weighing about 10½st, I started working as a childminder at a local crèche, where my weight was never an issue. But after a year working there, I received the shock of my life – I was pregnant! Amar was really supportive when I told him the news, and he took me out for a lovely meal to celebrate. That celebration meal marked the beginning of an all-out eating binge that lasted for nine months. All the clichés about 'eating for two' and 'needing to build up your strength' became my mantras. I wasn't big any more, I was pregnant – at last, I had an excuse to eat whatever I liked!

So what exactly did you eat?
I turned into a human Hoover, scoffing my way

BEFORE: *'I clocked all the slim beach babes and wished I was one of them'*

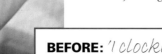

AFTER: *'I know I'm now one of those slim beach babes I've always admired'*

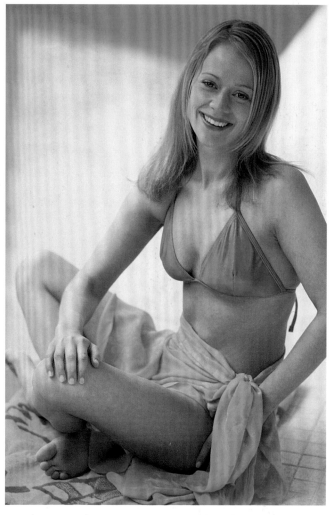

through loads of jam doughnuts in the middle of the night, and polishing off a huge bowl of Frosties in the morning. That would be followed by packets of biscuits, cakes, sausage rolls and ice cream as snacks during the day. For lunch, I would have a sandwich caked in butter, and then it was spaghetti bolognese for dinner, finished off with a sticky toffee pudding. On my 18th birthday, I managed to eat an entire chocolate cake on my own! My weight shot up to 12st, but I was sure that once the baby was born, the weight would drop off.

And did it?

No! Baby Aleicia arrived – but my bulge remained. I felt devastated, especially when I read about smug celebrity mothers who could fit into size 10-clothes only a few days after giving birth. It seemed that they lost the weight as if by magic, while I was left struggling with a massive spare tyre and zero motivation.

Did you try and lose the weight?

Even though I was depressed about my size, I just couldn't seem to do anything about it. Coming out of hospital after having Aleicia was just awful – everyone wanted to visit us, or for us to visit them. The trouble was, I couldn't fit into any of my pre-pregnancy clothes, and socialising in a shapeless smock wasn't an appealing prospect. I'd given up my job to be a full-time mum, and ended up spending the next two years at home, alone with

Aleicia – shovelling everything in sight into my mouth. Boredom played a big part in my bingeing, and I passed away the time by planning which of my favourite foods to eat next. Having a baby opens up a world that revolves around food. Every day, a friend would pop round for a chat, armed with cakes or packets of biscuits. It's amazing how quickly you can chomp your way through a packet of biscuits while chatting to your mates over a cup of tea. Before you know it, there goes another 1,000 calories down the hatch!

What was your turning point?

Amar, who works as a nightclub MC, was offered a booking for a few days in Ibiza in the summer of 2000, and the promoter asked if he would like to take me along on the trip. As soon as Amar told me, my heart hit the floor. The last thing I wanted to do was visit the party capital of Europe packed with beautiful people, while I was looking and feeling like a blob. Amar needed an on-the-spot decision from me. Unable to believe I was turning down an all-expenses paid trip abroad because I was ashamed of how I looked, I shook my head and told him 'no'. But as he walked off, something clicked inside me, and I ran after him shouting 'yes!' I was going to Ibiza, and I had five months to lose weight. Amar was delighted I was coming on the trip. He never mentioned my weight, but he was concerned about how I felt about myself and was supportive about my plan to get slim for the holiday.

How did you make a start?

I already knew about healthy eating – I just chose to ignore it! So, to inspire myself, I bought a copy of *Slimming* magazine, hoping it would set me on the straight and narrow. I couldn't be bothered with counting calories, but I cut right back on my fat intake. Soon, I was filling up on a couple of Weetabix with skimmed milk for breakfast. This was followed by a mid-morning fruit snack. For lunch, rather than slapping butter on my sandwich,

I'd use some Branston pickle to make it less dry. In the evening, I'd grill mushrooms and a piece of chicken, and add soy sauce for flavour. I also used soy sauce for cooking, rather than oil. I tried not to be too strict with myself – total denial usually ended with me caving in and eating even more. As a tasty low-fat treat, I'd chop up an apple, crush a caramel flavoured Snack-a-Jack into it, pour a toffee flavoured Müllerlight over the top, and add a sprinkling of raisins.

Did you brave the scales?

I certainly did. I made my weekly shopping trip to Boots my official weigh-in. The first time I weighed myself, I was mortified to see 11st 5lb flash up on the monitor – I had no idea I was that big. But that weighing machine, which also printed off a reading,

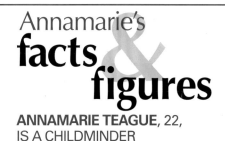

Annamarie's facts & figures

ANNAMARIE TEAGUE, 22, IS A CHILDMINDER

Height:	5ft
Weight then:	11st 5lb
Weight now:	7½st
WEIGHT LOST:	3st 12lb
Size then:	16
Size now:	8

turned out to be a real motivator. I stuck the first ticket onto the fridge door, to stop me raiding the fridge at night. After every weigh-in, I'd stick up my new ticket, and seeing the pounds drop off – at a rate of 1lb a week – became a real incentive.

Being a busy mum, was it difficult to find time to exercise?

Initially, I started swimming – and took Aleicia with me. The first time I went, I had to call ahead to make sure I would be allowed to wear shorts in the pool – I was far too embarrassed to don a swimming costume. But despite my apprehensions, it was fine, and no one batted an eyelid at me. When I got home, though, I burst into tears, because Aleicia had loved swimming so much. I couldn't believe I'd deprived her of so much fun, and had missed the sight of her happy face beaming from the water – just because I had a penchant for jam doughnuts and was too embarrassed to reveal my body in a swimming costume. From then on, I took Aleicia swimming at least once a week – and I ditched the shorts after the first couple of sessions.

I joined the local gym as well, and started going three evenings a week. On Saturday mornings, Amar would look after Aleicia while I spent an hour in the gym – then we'd swap over and I'd look after Aleicia while he went to the gym.

How did you stay motivated?

The feel-good factor is what did it for me – remembering how fantastic I felt after a workout spurred me on. Soon, I decided I wanted a bicycle for travelling to the gym and the shops. But when Amar bought me a bike, I found myself worrying that people would laugh at the sight of my ample behind perched on the seat! Once I realised that no one cared what I looked like, I drifted off into my own world as I cycled around – which was a great stress buster. It was a half-hour round cycle ride to and from the gym. Soon, I loved cycling so much that even when it was raining, I'd have to go out and get my cycling fix – having some 'me time' is such a lifesaver when you're a mum.

So did you get the beach body you wanted in time for Ibiza?

Not quite. I got down to just under 10st in time for the holiday. Being a size 14 meant that I could at

least feel comfortable in vest tops, but bikinis were still off limits. Walking down to the beach, I couldn't help clocking all the slim beach babes, and wishing I was one of them. But, after losing 1 ½st, I had so much more energy – and even though I wasn't exactly dancing on the podiums, I had a great time. Seeing all those beautiful girls in trendy clothes – and planning what outfits I would wear when I got to my target weight – gave me the inspiration to stick to my diet, and I lost 4lb during the holiday!

Was it all plain sailing from then on?

Not quite. I hit a plateau when I had about ½st still left to shift, and didn't lose any weight for about five months. I was quite happy with myself at that weight, but I still wanted to tone up a few wobbly bits. Then a friend suggested I try a spinning class, which involves high-energy speed cycling on an exercise bike. My sister and I decided to give it a go together, and I was amazed by how much I enjoyed it. The pumping music was motivating, and soon it became my favourite exercise. Best of all, it melted away the pounds. Because I still had by 'baby belly,' I also focused on toning my tummy and did 100 sit-ups a day, breaking them down into sets of 20, with a rest in between, to make them more manageable.

How did you feel when you finally reached your target weight?

I was shocked when, after nearly two years of dieting and exercising, I finally hit 7 ½st, a slim size 8. And, rather than stuffing my face to celebrate, I treated myself to some pampering goodies from The Body Shop. Being able to buy trendy clothes that I loved to wear, rather than settling for anything I could fit into, was amazing. At last, I was one of those well-dressed girls I'd admired, and could dance about and enjoy myself on a night out, instead of sitting on the sidelines feeling like a frump.

My family are really chuffed for me – they can see how much more energy I've got, and I can enjoy going shopping with my mum, instead of finding it a

depressing chore. Amar is thrilled, too – not with how I look, because he always loved me, whatever my weight – but with how happy I've become. When we went on a family holiday to Malta last October, I was full of beans, and couldn't wait to get out and enjoy myself. The best bit was being able to book a holiday and not be panic-stricken about having to lose weight in time, because I knew I was one of those slim beach babes I'd always admired. Knowing I looked – and felt – great in sarongs, shorts and a bikini was fantastic. But having the energy to run through the park with Aleicia is what I love the most about losing weight, and I just wish I'd done it sooner. Now I'm fit, slim and healthy, I really can make the most of being a mum.

Any plans for the future?

This summer I'm doing a 5km fun run to raise money for charity. I'm fitter than I've ever been, and still going to gym regularly, so I'm sure I'll manage it, no trouble.

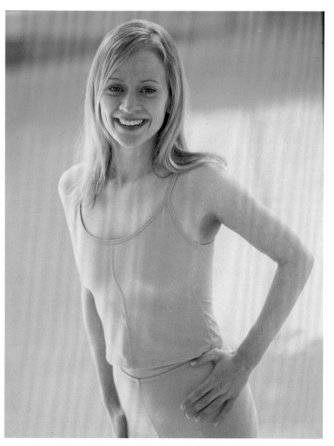

FEATURE: AMANDA ASTILL. PHOTOGRAPHY: RUTH JENKINSON. STYLING: MARIA ZOKAS. HAIR AND MAKE-UP: BRITTA D